Praise for *Taming Chronic Pain*

"Clear, engaging, and with the aut

—Patricia Morley-F
Professor Emerita, Western University
Former Director of Pain Management Program at Western University
Former Medical Director of Pain Management Program
at St Joesph's Hospital
2013 Canadian Anesthesiologists' Society Gold Medal Winner

"I would recommend this book to all chronic pain sufferers, family members, and doctors involved in managing chronic pain."

—Laxmaiah Manchikanti, MD, founder of *Pain Physician*

"An essential handbook for anyone who has to manage pain at some point in their life. And isn't that everyone?"

—Dr. Linda Clever, author of *The Fatigue Prescription*

"In this practical and empowering guide, Amy Orr offers hands-on strategies and insights that combine the wisdom and empathy of someone who has lived with pain with the clear-eyed precision of a skilled writer. *Taming Chronic Pain* is a concise yet comprehensive toolkit for living with—and moving beyond—chronic pain."

—Laurie Edwards, author of *Life Disrupted* and
In the Kingdom of the Sick
www.laurieedwardswriter.com

"Amy Orr has written a clear and persuasive primer on what it means to live with chronic pain. With a light, breezy style, she gives realistic advice on how to manage pain. No quack cures here; no shady fixes. Instead, you'll find useful tips on everything from how to talk to your doctor to knowing when to be weird (you'll understand when you read the book!). Relevant not only for people living with chronic pain, but also for those whose loved ones live in pain."

—Peter A. Ubel MD Professor of Medicine, Public Policy and Business Duke University Author of *Sick to Debt* (Yale, 2019) and *Critical Decisions* (HarperCollins)

"In *Taming Chronic Pain*, Amy Orr sets out to offer guidance and support to chronic pain patients in virtually every aspect of their lives, and she succeeds in her mission masterfully. As she writes: 'You are not your body but you are in your body, so it's your job to take care of it.' Orr helps every patient to do exactly that—sensibly, purposefully, and with optimism and good humor. She is frank in offering her advice or expertise, but without being preachy or didactic. Readers will come away feeling they have found a friend and valued advisor. I highly recommend *Taming Chronic Pain* and know that pain patients will benefit from reading it in many, many ways in their present and into their future."

—Joy H Selak PhD Author of *You Don't LOOK Sick! Living Well with Invisible Chronic Illness* with Dr. Steven Overman

TAMING CHRONIC PAIN

TAMING CHRONIC PAIN

A Management Guide
for a More Enjoyable Life

Amy Orr

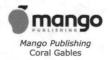

Mango Publishing
Coral Gables

Cover Design: Roberto Núñez
Layout & Design: Roberto Núñez
Illustrations by Jules Hall
Jules Hall is a Graphic Designer in Kitchener-Waterloo, where she lives with her partner and two cats. This book is close to her heart as she lives with chronic illness. If you're interested in seeing more of her work, visit juleshall.ca.

For permission requests, please contact the publisher at:
Mango Publishing Group
2850 S Douglas Road, 2nd Floor
Coral Gables, FL 33134 USA
info@mango.bz

For special orders, quantity sales, course adoptions and corporate sales, please email the publisher at sales@mango.bz. For trade and wholesale sales, please contact Ingram Publisher Services at customer.service@ingramcontent.com or +1.800.509.4887.

Taming Chronic Pain: A Management Guide for a More Enjoyable Life

Library of Congress Cataloging-in-Publication number: 2019941780
ISBN: (print) 978-1-64250-037-0, (ebook) 978-1-64250-038-7
BISAC category code: HEALTH & FITNESS / Pain Management

Printed in the United States of America

For little Amy.

The hardest lessons are learned with time.

Table of Contents

Part 2

Mind and Mood 90

Part 3

Tools and Therapies 138

Foreword

I was in the middle of a career as an anesthesiologist at a university teaching hospital in southwestern Ontario when I decided to go back to school. I wanted to learn more about chronic pain. I had been an obstetric anesthesiologist, relieving labor pain, and had also dealt with post-surgical pain in recovery and on the surgical floors. Surgical pain is acute pain. Doctors and nurses expect, understand, and know how to deal with acute pain. Usually what works for one patient after a certain surgery will work well to treat others after a similar surgery, with minor variations. But the world of chronic pain is very different, one problem being that what works for one person with a chronic pain condition might not work at all for someone with the same diagnosis. And the patient's life situation, mood, and past experience with pain are important in working toward pain control.

When I first started working in chronic pain clinics, I was struck by the lack of knowledge, scarcity of research, and general misconceptions around the condition of chronic pain. Here was a problem that one in five people in the United States and Canada suffer from, yet doctors-to-be received almost no training in it at any time in their undergraduate or postgraduate years.

Different medical specialties often held opposing views on how to assess and treat chronic pain. How could a patient experiencing the confusion, fatigue, and life-changing experience of chronic pain make sense of their problem if even their doctors couldn't? It is so multi-faceted and affects virtually every aspect of life, work, and relationships. Collaborative multi-disciplinary care for the patient, and education for the providers, seemed to make the most sense. Different approaches will appeal to different people.

Doctors do not come off well in *Taming Chronic Pain*, this recounting of author Amy Orr's journey of discovering how to live well with her chronic pain. I am happy to say that, in the past ten years, education in pain management has become mandatory in most Canadian and American medical schools. There is even a path to certification in the specialty of Pain Medicine now in Canada, as well as several other countries. In the future, I hope that patients reporting ongoing pain to their doctor will meet with fewer confused looks, and more understanding, than Amy did in her medical journey.

I was very pleased to be invited to write the foreword for this book. I first met Amy in 2014 when I was the medical director of the Multi-Disciplinary Pain Program at St. Joseph's Health Care in London, Ontario. To Amy, a curious person both by nature and training, this encounter was a revelation. The diagnosis gave a medical name to her sense of "feeling broken," and set her on the path to discovering everything she could about her condition. She has spent the last few years writing *Taming Chronic Pain* to explain all she has learned to others who are still trying to make sense of their own experiences.

It is unusual to find a book on chronic pain written by one who experiences it daily. When that person is also a writer and a scientist, the voice speaks confidently to a wide audience. This is not a book describing all current research on various pain disorders. It is a self-guided tour through the multiple aspects of causation, therapy, and self-awareness that an individual with chronic pain needs to understand in order to help themselves.

I was impressed by the work, woven out of Amy's personal experience and amplified by her thoughtfulness, curiosity, and research. Her style is candid about her own experiences and practical in her advice. The story reveals her struggles, but always guides the reader away from negativity to more positive feelings of choice and control.

Amy's writing style is conversational and direct, even blunt. Although easy to read, the information cannot all be digested, or applied, quickly. Many chapters end with a practical exercise, which should be read and worked on, time and again, in an effort to perfect the underlying skills they promote.

I think this book is useful for both patients and doctors. It deals with real concerns that clinicians and patients face. For example, I soon learned in the clinic that the available medications played a relatively small role in treatment. Side effects were frequent, the pain-relieving benefits small, and insurance coverage often difficult. In the long-term, self-management strategies play a greater role than medications alone. Many chapters here are devoted to aspects of self-management such as being aware of your personal energy ("Resource Management"), keeping moving ("Exercise and Pain"), and dealing with the inevitable anxiety and sadness ("Anxiety" and "Mindfulness and Meditation"). The chapter "Alternative Therapies" is the most practical guide that I have yet seen to sorting through available options. Interestingly to me, she recommends rating the therapies not necessarily on scientific evidence, rather on how they help the individual feel better.

In the introduction, and in the concluding summary, Amy makes it clear that there is no miracle cure. Rather the key to a better life with pain is to make small changes, little by little. And to become skilled at observing your body's response. This is the most important message of *Taming Chronic Pain*, told in such a way as to make it sound brand new. I only wish that I had this book available to me earlier so that I could have recommended it to my patients.

Patricia Morley-Forster, MD, FRCPC
Anesthesiology and Pain Medicine, Founder Status
Professor Emerita
Dept of Anesthesiology and Perioperative Care,
Western University, London, Canada
2013 Canadian Anesthesiologists' Society Gold Medal Winner

Getting Started

There Is No Miracle

Living your life while managing your pain—now there's a dangerous concept. For those who have experienced long-term chronic pain, this doesn't feel like an option. You can live your life, or you can manage your pain, but doing both together seems impossible. How can you go about your daily life if everything you do makes you hurt? How can you do what's best for your body without neglecting your life—your family, your job, your goals? Doing just one takes all the energy and strength you have. Believe me, I know this feeling well. It's either/or, and your body isn't giving you a lot of room to make the choice.

You don't, however, have to choose. It is possible to live your life and take care of your pain simultaneously, but it isn't easy and it isn't finite. It takes time and effort and will probably constantly change as the nature of your pain changes, as your life changes.

So, please, do not approach this book as *the answer*. I'm going to save you a lot of time by telling you there is no single answer. There is not a solution to chronic pain. What there is, is more complex: management techniques, behavioral changes, coping strategies, and support mechanisms that will make living with chronic pain easier, will make you better at adapting, will help your loved ones adapt and understand, and that can be practiced and molded over time. You can learn a wide variety of methods to deal with the physical, financial, emotional, and mental challenges of living with pain that develop and grow with you and your circumstances, and get you as close to the life you want as possible. That life may or may not be normal, it may or may not be what you originally wanted, and it will probably not be pain-free, but it will be easier. It will become an option for you to do both: live and manage your health.

I have spent many years living with chronic physical pain, and for a long time I didn't know that I was doing so. Doesn't everyone just hurt all the time? Isn't it normal to wake up exhausted after ten hours of sleep and be so stiff that you can't bend your knees or move your back? Everyone gets hurt! Everyone gets sick and has pain! So you do what people do: suck it up, ignore it, move on with your life. Denial gets us through tough times, but beware. Denial comes in many forms, but for many chronic pain sufferers it comes in the guise of "coping." Getting through each day, performing necessary tasks as best you can until your body gives out, gritting your teeth and plowing on ahead, despite how you feel—this is a form of denial. You are denying the reality of your body to get stuff done.

Don't get me wrong—this can be an effective strategy for some, for a short while. It often seems necessary. But in the long term, it has many flaws. For one, it will spectacularly blow up in your face the minute it is stress-tested. Because, if you're already living on the edge of what is possible for your body, when you are as healthy as you can be, what happens when you get a cold or break a bone or have to stay up through the night to meet a deadline? Or your kid gets sick, or you miss a meal, or any one of a million large and small things that happen to everyone all the time? You can't push any more, and stuff starts to slide.

Or, what happens when your body fights back against always being ignored? When the pain increases because you've been pushing through it and, again, you can't cope? Your life won't magically put itself on hold or restructure itself while you fix the problem. Denial is an extraordinarily powerful thing, but it can only last so long, and, when it's gone, the whole system collapses. And then you realize that you've spent your life coping rather than living.

I doubt anyone who has picked up a book titled *Managing Your Pain While Living Your Life* is still in this denial stage, but maybe you know someone who is. Maybe you lived there for a while yourself. Maybe you've still got one foot back there. There is no shame in that state; it is a natural emotional reaction to something that you cannot cope with. But this book is not intended for those living in that state or those who want a quick fix. Living and accepting a life with chronic pain is not for the faint of heart and, I'm sorry, it will require a lifetime of practice. But living can, absolutely, definitely, become easier.

I am not a doctor and I am not a miracle worker; I am not here to sell you snake oil or promise the unreasonable. I'm a scientist and professional problem-solver who has spent thirty years living with chronic pain disorders and the last ten studying them, researching tools and therapies for alleviation, and understanding the impact pain can have on every aspect of your life. Anyone who has been in long-term pain knows that this is not just about your body. Your mood, mental state, romantic relationships, financial situation, family, friends, career, hobbies, and life plans are all victims of pain—and that is the basis for this book.

There are a lot of books out there about living with chronic illness and living through pain—of many types. Many are excellent, and I have widely referenced plenty throughout this work; I encourage everyone to read as many as possible, do your own research, and listen to as many perspectives as possible. No two people's journeys will be the same; you probably already know that pain is individual, so having as much information as possible will provide you with a solid base from which to manage your own unique experience—which is why this book offers a little bit of everything. So, yes, we cover the science, the why— because understanding helps decrease the emotional suffering related to experiencing physical pain. Management techniques and practical suggestions are also here, in an effort to provide useful, actionable tools that can improve your life. And discussion of the emotional and mental effects pain can have on you and your family—because oftentimes, this is the worst part. This book may be whimsical or even silly at times, but that's okay. Pain isn't always rational, and we don't have to be, either. Part of my personal experience is that pain can make you a little crazy, and having a sense of humor about it is at times the only solution. We need to do whatever we need to do to make life's journey with pain as manageable as possible, for ourselves and our loved ones. But I guarantee, with work and time, you can get your freedom back and learn that pain does not have to dictate your life. Take heart, for others have been through what you are going through, and there is light at the end of the tunnel.

Part 1

THE BASICS

Chapter 1

Knowing Your Pain

I n order to get anywhere with your pain, you have to understand it. So let's start simple.

What Is Pain?

The nervous system runs throughout your body and sends electrochemical signals along its network of neurons, up the spine, and to the brain, where your brain interprets the signals it receives. The nervous system is the information highway for pain, but it is not the neurons themselves that "feel" the pain—your brain is what receives the information and draws your awareness to the part of the body that sent the signal. The central nervous system is an incredibly complex, highly developed system whose main purpose is to send messages between different parts of your body—from one cell to another. Pain is just one of these signals; when a part of you hurts, a signal is sent from the sensory receptors at that site, along the neural network to the brain, where the message "pain" is received and interpreted.

Pain serves many functions, but its most basic is to alert you, your consciousness, that something is wrong and a response is required. The response may be simple and reflexive (take your hand out of the fire), or even unconscious (causing your glands to secrete hormones to counteract the situation). Adrenaline may be released. Your body may tense up. Inadvertent and complex results may and do occur as the result of physical pain. But the thing you need to remember is: pain is there to help you. It warns you when something is wrong, makes sure you know to protect yourself. It is a valuable evolutionary tool.

But that is not to say it is infallible. Pain can be misleading. Your brain does not always interpret pain correctly and your sensory receptors do not always receive information accurately. There are many ways your body can fail you when it comes to pain, and one of the most common is for pain to be of a greater magnitude, of a longer duration, or simply from an insignificant cause, leading your brain to overreact and you to feel much more pain than is appropriate.

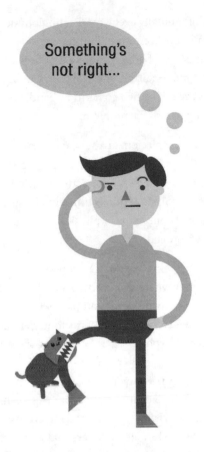

Broadly speaking, there are three traditional classifications of pain: acute, chronic non-cancer, and chronic cancer pain. While all pain is painful, not all pain is equal or behaves in the same way. Those who experience chronic pain feel changing effects over time, as their nervous system reacts to the environment of ongoing pain. In this way, acute pain is very different, and while they may be hard to differentiate in any given instant, chronic and acute pain are treated differently. Note, however, that acute pain can transition to chronic pain over time.

We're not going to delve into all of the various pain disorders here, as there are many, and even the same disorders can have different effects on different people. There are also many types of non-physical pain, and this is where life can get really complicated, because emotional pain and physical pain are not mutually exclusive. Feeling physically crappy can cause a negative emotional response. Feeling anxious or overwhelmed or depressed, or any number of other negative emotions, can cause physical symptoms of pain. Emotional and physical pain can become a self-reinforcing vicious cycle. The two go hand in hand, and pretending they don't means ignoring half of the problem.

Diagnosing and treating emotional pain is an enormous task and one that should, ideally, be tackled with the help of professionals. Later in this book, we will look at some of the specific emotional consequences of physical pain, but the analysis of *purely* emotional issues is not our target here. We want to narrow our focus to physical pain and its consequences, some of which are emotional.

So let's look at physical pain in depth. Do you know what type of pain you have? Do you know where it's coming from or what's causing it? That can be a simple question to answer if you have a broken leg or a burned hand, and these are relatively easy problems to understand and treat, but it's much tougher for amorphous pain. One of the most fundamental techniques you need to master, as a starting point for everything else, is understanding your pain. Know it, label it. This is not a one-step process. Your pain may well change over time. You need to be able to bring your awareness to whatever hurts, objectively assess it, and respond appropriately. You have to be able to depersonalize it, every time.

So what's your pain like? Let's break it down into some simple components and descriptors.

Classifying Pain

Duration

Acute Pain

Acute pain is typically sudden, intense, and short-lived. It is an immediate reaction to stimuli and is usually solved (or greatly ameliorated) by medical intervention.

Chronic Pain (Non-Cancer)

Chronic non-cancer pain is longer-lasting, often duller, and resistant to medical treatment. It can be linked to a physical or mental illness (other than cancer) but is not necessarily defined by it and can far outlast the original illness. The official definition of chronic pain is pain that lasts more than three months, and this definition can therefore encompass anything from prolonged recovery from injury to long-term illness.

Chronic Pain (Cancer)

Chronic cancer pain is long-term pain caused directly by cancer. Most cancer pain is caused by a tumor pressing on a nerve, bone, or organ. It can also be a result of cancer treatment—for example, pain experienced due to chemotherapy.

Breakthrough Pain

Breakthrough pain isn't technically its own category, as it's a form of pain that occurs when an ongoing chronic pain problem suddenly becomes acute—but we've kept it separate here because it does behave differently than chronic or acute pain. Breakthrough pain is often caused by a change or failure in medications, and although it is a function of the chronic pain, it acts and feels acute. This is most common among patients who are under treatment and have bouts of severe pain that break through their medication at intervals.

Location

Localized Pain

Most pain stays where it was caused; you break a leg, your leg hurts. You get stung by a bee on your finger, your finger hurts. Localized pain stays at its origin site.

Referred Pain

Referred pain is when pain from one part of your body is felt somewhere else.

Phantom Pain

Phantom pain is where there is pain in a part of the body that has been removed.

Intensity

Traditionally, pain is rated on a simple scale, from one to ten, depending on how it feels to you.

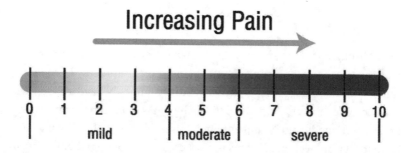

Mild Pain

A rating of one on the scale is effectively no pain at all. Anything between one and four is considered mild pain and can be ignored or easily treated.

Moderate Pain

Moderate pain is a five or six on the scale; it hurts, and you know it hurts, but it's not blotting out rational thought or your basic functionality.

Severe Pain

Severe pain is anything from a seven to a ten on the scale. If one is no pain at all, ten is the worst pain you have ever experienced. A ten on the scale is mind-numbing, searing, extreme pain that blocks basic functions such as walking or even breathing.

Note that, although we have split the pain scale up here to illustrate the range of severity, these are not different *types* of pain—just different *levels*. A pain of intensity one on the scale may behave exactly like a pain of intensity ten; it's just that the effect on you is different.

Pain Inventory

Many clinics now use a more sophisticated methodology than the simple one-to-ten pain scale. While helpful in acute situations (like in a hospital's emergency room), the one-to-ten scale doesn't reflect the changing nature and effects of chronic pain. Almost all chronic pain clinics use some form of pain inventory, pain interference, or pain functionality system to measure pain's severity and effect, as well as the effectiveness of treatments.

These systems may vary slightly by clinic and region, but, essentially, they record the pain at its high and its low, and the level of disruption the pain causes in key areas of life, such as sleep, work, mood, etc. This gives a better overall illustration of pain and how it impacts daily life on an ongoing basis, and doctors can use these systems to find ways to reduce the impact of the pain (even when they can't change the pain itself).

Cause

Pain is often classified by the damage that causes it, and there are layers of classification, depending on how in-depth you want to get. Let's look at them, starting with the broadest terms:

Nocioceptive Pain

Nocioceptive pain is a fancy way of saying pain from any of the physical structures of your body. This can include organs, muscles, skin, joints, and tissues.

Neuropathic Pain

This is the type of pain caused by damage to or a disease of the nervous system itself; it can affect any area of the body and can come in many forms: a stabbing pain, an ache, a shock, tingling or numbness, a burning sensation, a spasm. It can be continuous or episodic. Neuropathic pain is notoriously hard to treat and often is the most persistent, least understood of all types of pain.

Algopathic or Central Sensitization Pain

This is pain caused by the brain's perception of the sensations reaching it. It is not a function of the physical body, the tissues, joints, muscles, organs, or even the central nervous system, but rather is caused by neurological disorders that affect the way the brain interprets information.

These three basic types of pain are the main classifications.[1] But we can go down a level into different types of pain:

Visceral Pain

Visceral pain is associated with injury to the internal organs and is usually acute until the underlying illness is treated.

Somatic Pain

This is the most common form of everyday pain, affecting sensory receptors within the muscles, soft tissues, or skin. Examples of somatic pain are mild burns, muscular inflammation, an insect bite.

Psychogenic Pain

Psychogenic pain refers to physical pain that is caused by psychological factors only, with no physical cause component. This is extremely rare. Mood can magnify pain in many ways, but very rarely does it cause pain all on its own

And going further still into specific types of pain within the body:

Joint Pain, Bone Pain, Muscular Pain, Nerve Pain

Rather obviously, these labels refer to a specific type of body part that is affected by pain. If you pull a muscle, you have muscular pain. If you have arthritis or another illness affecting the joints, you have joint pain. If you have a broken bone or a form of bone disease, this is bone pain. Or, if you have nerve damage, this causes nerve pain. These are simple classifications, but you probably already know the feel of each one—most of us have pulled a muscle in our time or overdone it and had a sore back.

---

1   Clifford J Woolf, *Classifications of Pain.*

Sensations

There are a lot of different ways that pain can *feel*. No two people experience pain identically, and you are the only person who is feeling the pain that you're feeling. No one else can tell you how it feels. It is important that you can name your pain, describe it, and distance yourself from it. Not only will this help you to understand it, describe it to your doctor, identify what is happening in your body, and analyze your possible responses, but it will also help distance you from it emotionally. You are not your pain, and your pain does not define you. Try imaging your pain as a really unwelcome, disliked family member you simply cannot get rid of.

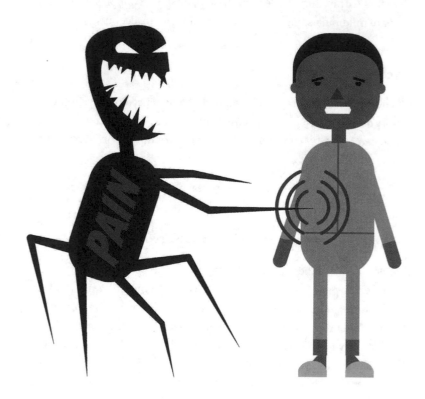

Here are some helpful words that you can use to describe the feel of your pain(s):

spasm	tingling	episodic	stinging	raw
aching	numb	persistent	searing	thumping
dull	itching	irritant	lwinge	tight
sharp	burning	tickling	cramp	pressure/vise-like
acute	cold	prickling	tenderness	mild
stabbing	shock	throbbing	inflamed	intense
pounding	radiating	boring	pinching	pulsing
rasping	grinding	swollen	lacerating	nagging

Common Causes of Chronic Pain

Chronic pain can be anything that lasts longer than three months, but some chronic pain ailments are permanent and others are, ultimately, temporary. There are many different illnesses that can cause chronic pain; below are just some of the most common. Even these can come with complications, comorbidities and unusual presentations, so this is not intended to be an exhaustive or prescriptive list—just a rough guide to the most widely diagnosed chronic pain ailments at present.

Arthritis

Arthritis is the most common cause of pain, affecting almost one in every two adults over the age of sixty-five. Arthritis is not simply a disease of the elderly, however, with over a third of working-age adults experiencing it in some form at some point in their lives. Arthritis affects the joints through inflammation and can make movement painful.

Chronic Back Pain

According to research, almost 85 percent of adults will experience chronic back pain at some point. This may be due to injury, accident, arthritis, or through normal wear and tear, but anyone who has suffered this particular issue knows it can be immobilizing and very difficult to treat. It is rare for chronic back pain to become permanent.

Fibromyalgia

Fibromyalgia affects the nervous system and is associated with widespread pain in the muscles and bones without apparent cause. It can cause severe fatigue and general bodily tenderness, as well as cognitive impairment. It is the second most common condition affecting bones and muscles but, because of its amorphous symptoms, is often misdiagnosed.

Psychogenic Pain Disorder

Pain problems associated with psychological factors only, without physical cause, are known as psychogenic disorders. They can be caused by stress, anxiety, depression, or mood disorders and can present as headaches, migraines, back pain, stomach pain, or muscular pain. Given the wide range of possible affected areas, psychogenic pain is usually diagnosed when all potential physiological causes have been ruled out.

Chronic Headaches

Headaches are commonplace, but some people suffer from headaches which last at least fifteen days per month, for consecutive months, thereby becoming officially *chronic*. These can be tension headaches, migraines, cluster headaches, or eye-related headaches, but are exhausting and debilitating, whatever the cause.

Sciatica

Sciatica occurs when the sciatic nerve, the largest peripheral nerve in the body, running from your spine down your leg, becomes irritated. This is most common among patients with a herniated spinal disc but can also occur due to accident or other injury. Symptoms include electric-shock-like pain down the leg, numbness and tingling, and muscle weakness. Sciatica can be persistent unless the root cause of the problem is addressed.

All pain is personal, because it's happening to you, but that does not mean it *is* you. As we've seen in this chapter, pain is an evolutionary tool that can and does get out of hand, but that doesn't mean you are lacking in control. Sun Tzu advises us to "know your enemy,"[2] so become acquainted with your pain. Give it a silly name if it helps. Talk to it. Scold it. Describe it. How can you expect to live with it if you don't take the trouble to get to know it?

---

2   Sun Tzu, *The Art of War*.

Exercise:
Know Your Pain

One of the most helpful tools you can use to understand your pain and to help your caregivers understand is to create your own pain profile. This can seem like a lot of work, but once you are practiced at it, it will become second nature and allow you to objectively understand what you are feeling and what, if anything, you need to do about it.

Start by keeping a simple pain diary. Every day, record the following *for each individual pain* you can identify:

- Location of pain

- Duration of pain

- Intensity of pain

- Description of pain

- Activity immediately before pain

- Medications or action taken for pain and their effect

You can use the list of descriptive words shown earlier to narrow down the feeling of the pain you are experiencing. It is vital that you are able to perceive how your pain manifests and its effect on your day and your world.

Performing this exercise while in pain can be tough, but do the best you can. It may be easier for you to wait until the end of the day, and record every instance you can remember at once—this also helps you to separate and categorize different types of pain you have felt through the day.

Chapter 2

Talking to Your Doctor

Talking to your doctor about, well, anything, can be tough.
Embarrassing, strained, rushed, complicated. Even the simplest
problem can be difficult to talk about with someone who may well be
almost a stranger. But here's the thing: you cannot afford to treat your
doctor as a stranger. Yes, you may have only met him/her a few times.
Yes, you may not like them very much. But you need to be able to give
them detailed, personal information so they can help you as best they can.
There is no avoiding this. No one can do it for you, and, if you don't do it,
it won't get done. A doctor will not magically guess the right treatment for
you. It's up to you to give him or her all of the relevant information.

In the last chapter we said that pain was not infallible. Well, guess what?
Neither is your doctor. Unless you are reading this from an incredibly
privileged position of wealth, the overwhelming likelihood is that your
doctor is overworked, underpaid, stretched across too many patients, and
working without enough sleep, support, or resources to properly help his
or her patients. Appointment time varies by country, but the average is
just over ten minutes—significantly less for more than half of the world's
population (eighteen countries have appointment times of less than five
minutes), and a little more for wealthier nations (twenty minutes in the
USA).[3] Imagine that. Ten minutes—including prescreening by a nurse or
medical assistant—to have an in-depth discussion with your doctor about
your symptoms, possible causes, and treatment options and to think of
and ask intelligent follow-up questions. That's a tall order even for the
most self-assured, articulate person.

---

3   Carolyn Crist, "The doctor will see you now—but often not for long," Reuters, last modified November
     28, 2017, https://www.reuters.com/article/us-doctor-checkup-duration/the-doctor-will-see-you-now-but-
     often-not-for-long-idUSKBN1DS2Z2.

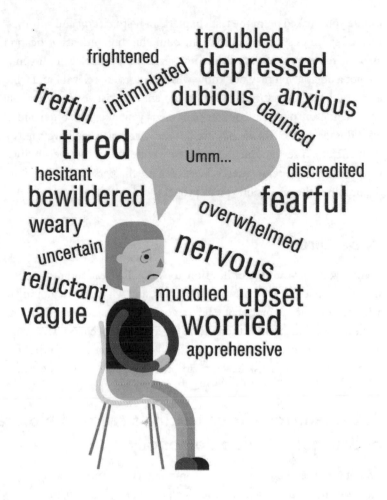

So What Can I Do?

1. Be Prepared

This is the one best single, practical thing you can do to ensure your appointment is productive and your health care provider is put in the best position to help you. Before you attend your appointment, write down everything you need to say. List your symptoms (this is where the pain profile you worked on in the last chapter can help) clearly and simply. Include specifics such as nature of the pain, duration, intensity, location, associated factors—even if you are not sure if they are relevant. If you are not a doctor, you may not know which factors are relevant and which aren't, so let your doctor make that judgment call. List your medications and include any over-the-counter pain meds you take, how often and what dosage, how effective they are. List any therapies you have tried and their efficacy. If serious, include effects on your mood, routine, ability to work, sex drive, appetite, exercise, etc. You are the person experiencing the problem; the onus is on you to properly describe it.

2. Be Direct

Neither you nor your doctor has time to waste. Be clear and direct about why you have come in, what the problem is, and what you are hoping to achieve from the appointment. Have a goal in mind: a new medication, suggestions for alternative therapies, a referral to a specialist. This may or may not end up being the result, but if you do not have an intention for the appointment, you risk leaving without having made any progress.

3. Do Not Take Your Doctor's Harried Nature or Brusque Attitude Personally

Do not interpret their attitude as a commentary on your medical situation. Your health care provider is a person, just like you, not a magical all-knowing being with endless capacity for patience and kindness. We might want them to be that, but they're not. If they're having a crappy day, they may well show it. Don't personalize that. If it's bad, if you feel they're not listening to you, say so. You are allowed to do that! You have come in with a potentially tricky, difficult-to-diagnose-or-treat problem, and you should have their full attention.

4. Consider Asking for More Time

Pain is a complicated issue, and it is reasonable to expect a discussion of it to take longer than that of a cold or a sprained ankle. When making your appointment (especially with a general practitioner), consider asking for a longer appointment or an appointment at the end of the day—tell the receptionist you feel you need more time to speak with your doctor. They may not be able to help you, but most will appreciate your desire to avoid messing up their schedule by running long in the middle of the day.

5. Ask for a Referral

You may not be able to get the help you need from your family doctor or a specialist for a specific illness. Chronic pain specialists exist and focus purely on the understanding and treatment of physical pain. They have a wealth of knowledge your regular doctor does not and can be valuable resources. Consider asking your doctor for a referral, if this is an option near you.

6. Take Notes during Your Appointment

This may feel silly, but you probably have a lot of doctors' appointments, regularly, and keeping track of it all can be an important diagnostic and treatment tool. Writing down your doctors' suggestions, medication advice, and thoughts prevents you from forgetting anything, helps clear up confusion about instructions, and will strengthen the dialogue between you.

7. Take Suggestions Seriously

Your doctor may suggest a medication or treatment that you are uncomfortable with. You are well within your right to say so at the time— but do not discount everything. Doing so will discourage your doctor from trying to problem-solve with you and leave you even more on your own. Take their advice on board and, if possible, take notes on what you have tried and its efficacy.

Your relationship with your doctor is a partnership and should be treated as such. They are not gods who can wave their hands and solve every problem, but neither are you. You can and should demand time, attention, and respect from your doctor and for your pain, but do so realizing that they, like you, may be doing their best to fix an unfixable problem. It is your responsibility to be your own advocate for your health.

Misunderstanding Pain

Pain is a deeply misunderstood issue, and it can be very difficult to get a health care professional to take you seriously. All too often, we hear, "I told my doctor about the pain, but he said it was normal" or, "She said everyone gets that, I just have to suck it up and deal with it like everyone else." Yes, everyone experiences pain at one time or another. And yes, it is all too common for doctors to try to explain pain away as a temporary symptom of something else, or even imaginary. The most heard (and most offensive) phrase for chronic pain sufferers is "It's all in your head." This dismissiveness and ignorance make a formal diagnosis incredibly difficult to come by. Those of you who have one probably had to see multiple doctors, maybe over a long period of time, before you were taken seriously.

Unfortunately, this is a problem that disproportionately affects women, who are perceived as having a lower pain tolerance and being more prone to complaint. This is simply false, and any doctor who tries to dismiss your legitimate pain for any reason, let alone gender, is wasting your time.

Not being taken seriously is the number one complaint those with pain disorders register when dealing with the medical profession. This is not necessarily anyone's fault—an overworked, stressed doctor who has seen twenty people in a row with trifling complaints may be dismissive by habit rather than through callousness—but it does affect you, your health, and the management of your pain. Your pain is not secondary to your doctor's mood (or timekeeping), and the single most effective way to ensure it is not treated as such is by not letting it be.

Sounds easy, right? Sure, I won't let it. I'll just snap my fingers and hey! presto, the doctor will take me seriously. And when the doctor I've been waiting three months to see dismisses my pain with a wave of his hand and declares I'm just "being dramatic," I won't take it personally and collapse into tears, thereby validating his assumption that I'm overly emotional or attention-seeking. I'll be completely stoic, an emotionless robot who ignores her pain as callously as the doctor in front of me does.

Well, no. Expecting heroic displays of objectivity from ourselves, or high levels of compassion from every doctor, will lead to disappointment. But you can say, "I don't think you're taking me seriously." Call them on it. See how they respond. Or, how about: "Here is a list of recent instances of pain, with extensive details of intensity, duration, et cetera. I would appreciate it if you tried to hear what I'm telling you, and I thought this list would help you understand." Make it their problem—they were clearly unable to understand you the first time, so you've provided an idiot's guide. Or how about simply: "This is not a problem I am willing to walk out of here without solving."

These are difficult things to say. We are taught to respect our doctors, to listen to them, to defer to them. Being your own advocate is not easy and may not always make you friends. But what's your alternative? Bow your head, nod, agree, and leave with the problem unsolved? It's okay, I'll just keep using this medication that does nothing. It's alright, I can live with this pain by myself with no medical support. If you think that's a realistic option, you may not be ready to call bullshit on your doctor. That's okay—a lot of people aren't. But don't expect improvement, or for your pain to become manageable by itself, if so. Know the decision you are making.

In the vast majority of cases, calling them out is an extremely effective way of capturing your health care professional's attention and ensuring they listen to you. They still may not be able to help—but at least you're not screaming into the void. And for those doctors—and there are some—who are simply unwilling to believe you, walk away. Nothing can be achieved by seeing them again. How are you supposed to trust them with your health if they so clearly don't trust you?

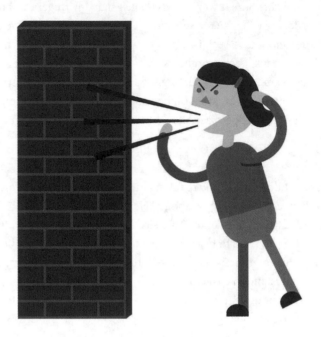

Misinformation

Misinformation about pain abounds, not just among medical professionals, but also online and in the media. So another important aspect of your self-advocacy is educating yourself. Even the best, most compassionate doctor can't know everything. There may be options out there for you that they are unaware of; there may be practical solutions or advice that will help; you may even occasionally be told something that's just flat-out not true. You need access to as much helpful and accurate data as possible, and you need to be able to spot the fiction. Be prepared to do your own research: visit forums, do internet searches, read books and health websites, and talk to other people with similar pain issues. There is a wealth of valuable information out there, and while it may not feel like it's your job to find it, you are the person who'll suffer if you don't.

The Doctor's Role

So we've said quite a few things already about doctors not listening, rushing, or not believing you. This is true in some cases, and may *feel* true in many more, but in order for you to really appreciate what you can expect from your doctor and know how to manage your relationship with your doctor, let's look at their perspective for a second.

Until very recently, medical students were not trained in diagnosing, managing, or communicating chronic pain issues. It simply wasn't in the curriculum. This has been rectified, and now all new doctors trained in North America have at least some tools to understand and explain chronic pain, but older doctors may not. They are the victims of changing standards, and probably perceive their responsibility toward you very differently than you do. Be aware of this, and allow this knowledge to prevent you from taking your doctor's apparent attitude too personally.

It's also important to know what a doctor is looking for and what a doctor is typically asked for, when a patient presents with chronic pain. Broadly speaking, there are three main issues:

1. First, the doctor must determine that the pain is not indicative of a new problem. Chronic pain sufferers can still get injuries and illnesses, and the doctor must satisfy himself or herself that nothing new or potentially threatening is happening before they address the known, chronic problem. Don't get angry if your doctor seems to be re-treading old ground every time you visit— they're not ignoring you or failing to listen; they're safeguarding against something worse.

2. Imaging requests. Patients typically overestimate the usefulness of
    imaging techniques in diagnosing and treating chronic illnesses.
    An MRI or an ultrasound may sound like something that will give
    you answers and help you, but, in reality, they may be useless. Do
    not assume that a doctor who refuses to order certain tests is not
    taking you seriously. And, if you're really concerned about a lack
    of tests, ask your doctor to put in your medical record the reasons
    they won't order any. If they have a valid reason, then fine—if not,
    this can often spur them to action.

3. Medications are sometimes thought of as the answer to everything.
    We'll discuss medication types and addiction issues later in the
    book—and clearly the over-prescription of strong painkillers is a
    difficult and complex issue—but again, refusal to prescribe certain
    meds is not necessarily a reflection on you or on your doctor's
    belief in your pain. Doctors are facing pressure (and research
    supports that pressure) to lay off strong painkillers (especially
    opioids) and work with patients in pursuing alternative pain
    relief options. This trend will absolutely affect how your doctor
    interacts with you.

None of this is to say that there aren't some doctors who dismiss chronic
pain, belittle the need for extra help or meds, or ignore requests for
disability paperwork support. Of course there are—most of us have met at
least one of these doctors at some point—but not every harried, put-upon
or poorly trained doctor is out to get you personally. For a more in-depth
understanding of the divide in expectations and comprehension that
influences communication issues between patients and doctors, I can do
no better than recommending a book by Peter Ubel, MD: the excellent
Critical Decisions. This book brilliantly covers what patients can expect—
and what is expected of them—when working with a physician.

What You Will and Won't Get

What to Expect from Your Doctor

- Time
- Attention
- Takes you seriously
- Asks questions
- Takes notes
- Recommends possible treatment options
- A referral if appropriate, with expected wait times
- Prescriptions

What You'll Probably Get from Your Doctor

- A little time, but not enough
- Some questions, some of which you may not see the relevance of
- Confirmation of medications
- Suggestions of treatments and therapies
- Possible confusion (especially if they're not trained in chronic pain)
- A statement that pain is tricky and they cannot be certain what is going on

What Your Doctor Can Expect from You

- Honesty
- Respectful attitude

- An honest, up-front assessment of what you can and cannot manage, given your lifestyle

- An open mind

- Awareness that they are working to a certain mandate and under certain restrictions

Things You Didn't Know You Could Say to Your Doctor

- "I would like another doctor."

- "I would like a referral."

- "This prescription has bad side effects: I need another."

- "You are not listening to me," or "I feel as if you're not listening to me."

- "This is not a normal pain and I need you to recognize that."

- "This is causing serious problems in my life, and I need you to help me."

- "Your behavior is making me anxious, and I am unable to continue with this appointment."

- "I need to come back another time."

- "Please give me a moment; this is difficult to talk about."

Know Your Rights

Each country and each medical system is different, so this is a tough topic—especially if you have transitioned from one system to another because of a relocation or financial change. But it is extremely important to know your rights as a patient, under the law, wherever you are. The law and medical governing bodies will set out a wide range of influencing factors in your health care, including: data protection, privacy, complaint procedures, extent of financial coverage, extent of financial liability, doctors' required qualifications, medical practice insurance requirements, your medical insurance requirements, access to care (both primary and ongoing), and a million other things. Your ability to pay, ask for a referral or a new doctor, lodge a complaint, see your own records, or pursue alternative treatment avenues will all depend on your particular medical system. So research it. Know your rights—it will put you in a much stronger position when discussing your health care with your providers.

Exercise:
Making Notes for Your Doctor's Appointment

Making notes for a medical appointment is an important skill. Before your next discussion with your doctor, try the following:

1. Write down, in any format you like, everything you wish to discuss.

2. Under each topic, list the symptoms you are concerned about.

3. Under each symptom, write as much detail as you can about it. Include medications, treatments, and any other factors (lifestyle and otherwise) that you think may be affecting it.

4. Under that, write down how this symptom affects your day and give it a seriousness rating from one to ten.

5. Finally, read back through your notes. Are they clear? If not, try organizing them. Have a planned order in mind to frame your upcoming discussion, and set out your notes in that order.

6. List your questions at the end.

7. Consider typing up brief, bullet-pointed notes to give to your doctor during your appointment—this may save time for you both and will give them something to reference.

Example

Symptom 1	Symptom 2	Symptom 3	Symptom 4
Any meds used	Any meds used	Any meds used	Any meds used
Any treatments	Any treatments	Any treatments	Any treatments
Factors affecting this	Factors affecting this	Factors affecting this	Factors affecting this
Seriousness 1–10	Seriousness 1–10	Seriousness 1–10	Seriousness 1–10
Description of its effect	Description of its effect	Description of its effect	Description of its effect

Question 1:

_____

_____

_____

Question 2:

_____

_____

_____

Question 3:

_____

_____

_____

Chapter 3

Age, Gender, and Pain

A small note about pain as it relates to some basic aspects of you: firstly, age. It is a well-known fact that, as we age, our bodies deteriorate, and once-simple tasks may become painful or even unachievable. That is a normal and expected part of life. However, the rate at which we deteriorate can vary widely, and, for those of us who have chronic health problems from a young age, the process starts earlier and can proceed more swiftly than average.

While many aspects of pain management apply to the expected symptoms of aging—such as arthritis—there is an aspect of pain management that the young have to perform, that the elderly do not. The fetishism of youth (a.k.a. health) makes it much, much harder for younger sufferers of chronic pain to live openly managing their pain. There is an awful phrase that I'm sure many, many of you have heard: "Well, you look fine." Ah, of course. I look fine, therefore I must be fine. I am only twenty, or thirty, or forty, so by your standards there really can't be anything much wrong with me. I must be exaggerating. I must be lazy, or a hypochondriac. There are no physical symptoms like a cast on my leg, and I am not eighty and therefore immune from your judgment about my health, ergo everything is well. This is, sadly, an opinion that even some doctors profess—if they can't find anything wrong with you on first examination, then there is nothing wrong. Pull yourself together. Only the elderly experience physical deterioration.

Sadly, younger sufferers of pain do not experience camaraderie with others—friends in a similar physical state—or shared understanding of the world at large. It would be patently wrong to hurry along an elderly person in front of you on the sidewalk, but doing this to a younger person is socially acceptable. And complaining about a sore hip may be normal for a seventy-year-old, but being twenty and doing this makes you a whiner. No, it's not fair.

It's easy to look at those attitudes in the abstract and know they are wrong, know that those judgmental people don't know you, don't know that you are doing the best you can. But knowing that and feeling that way in the face of bemused stares and probing questions are two very different things. We will talk later about shoulding and its negative effects. There is a very difficult, specific part of shoulding that happens only to the young,

and it is all-encompassing: *you should be healthy*. The fundamental belief
that ill-health only comes with age is a pernicious and dangerous one
and leads many people to ignore or try to tough their way through pain,
without ever understanding the cause or becoming able to make it better.
Again, knowing that someone is doing this to you is a very different thing
from being able to say so, or being able to recognize it in the moment.
More often than not, even for the most rational and self-assured people
out there, the exclamation "You look fine!" will make you want to prove
it, to live up to that, to agree and minimize and stop putting your pain
management first. There is no amount of life experience that can stop this
from happening, but you can stop it from affecting how you manage your
health. Shame is a natural result of someone trying to shame you, but
don't let it change the way you have decided, rationally and calmly and
with your doctor, to act. Someone else's judgment is not more important
than your need to manage yourself.

A similar point exists for gender and pain. Socially, there is an
understanding that "men are tougher," "real men don't cry," and other
similarly asinine expectations that can make living in pain, openly, very
difficult for men. Why don't you just man up? Tough your way through
it? Real men don't let pain stop them. This is such obvious nonsense in
the abstract that it's hard to even write down, but it's a very real aspect
of many chronic pain sufferers' lives that can make seeking treatment,
accepting help, or even discussing their bodies with loved ones much
harder. And, as with age, there is not really a way to stop this happening,
to prevent society at large from putting these expectations on you. All you
can do is make sure you are taking thoughtful care of yourself, follow your
doctor's advice, speak up when you feel able to challenge the nonsense,
and ignore it when you don't. Remember, your body is more important
than other people's expectations.

A Note on Exhaustion

A hidden but significant aspect of living with pain is exhaustion. This comes in several forms, the simplest of which is the basic feeling of being physically and mentally tired from just existing. Getting through each day takes a toll, being in pain is hard, and many people are understandably dog-tired at the end of it. Your overall energy is lower when you experience pain, and this is true for everyone, regardless of age or gender.

Sleep is a separate but also very important issue for chronic pain sufferers. Getting quality sleep is much harder when in pain, when battling the side effects of medications, and when anxious about health. The normal consequences of living with pain lead to lack of sleep, and this massively contributes to physical and mental exhaustion. Many pain sufferers even suffer from chronic insomnia. The ability to rest effectively is crucial to allowing the body and brain time to recover, and, without this, pain is compounded. This is a perfect example of a vicious circle: in pain, can't sleep, more pain (because you're tired), can't sleep.

Even the youngest or toughest person can quickly become fatigued when living with pain, and this presents many challenges to going about your daily life. Unfortunately, the solution is simple yet difficult: you have to put your rest first. First, no exceptions. No excuses. If what you need to rest effectively is to take a nap every afternoon, then that's what you have to do. I don't care if you're twenty-five or seventy-five. You need sleep and rest, whatever this looks like for you, whatever anyone else thinks. Rest is one of the single most important tools in pain management. If it means a special soft bed, then great. If it means sleeping with a prop, go for it. If it means going to bed at eight o'clock and not getting to bar-hop with friends, then this is the decision you have to make. If you do not prioritize your body's need to rest, you are not prioritizing your health. Fatigue is potentially deadly, so be proactive and don't let it get on top of you.

Exercise:
Seeing Through Age and Gender

Compassion toward yourself takes practice. Start trying to exercise compassion toward others. If someone is walking slowly on the street, don't just hurry past them. Think to yourself: maybe that's as fast as they can walk. Ignore their age or the way they look. If someone can't lift a bag of groceries at the market, don't think "They're weak" or "They should exercise more." Think: maybe they're experiencing muscular difficulty today. Maybe their joints have seized up.

Being in pain can feel like being on an island alone, and this fosters an *everyone else* mentality. It seems like everyone else can cope fine, has no issues, has their good health. But pain is invisible; just as they don't know yours, you don't know theirs. Stop presuming about others' bodies and pain, and it will become easier to stand up for your own.

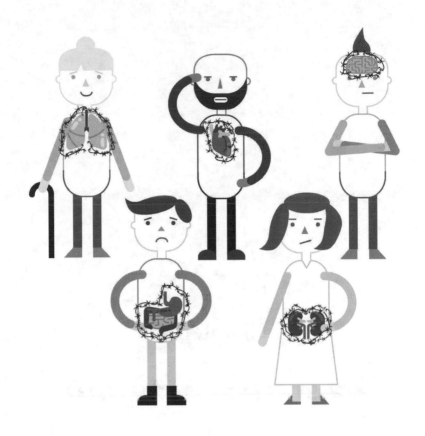

Chapter 4

Exercise and Pain

The room is full of oddly shaped, baffling apparatus with shelves and seats and levers and switches and buttons and ropes and pedals and weights and platforms and oh my God, what are you supposed to do with that bar?

Gyms are intimidating—sometimes by design. A lot of people learn how to use a piece of exercise equipment by surreptitiously watching someone else use it. A lot, more simply, join a sports team, or cycle or run by themselves, or find a class, or simply don't bother.

We all know that exercise is good for us and that most doctors recommend a minimum of thirty minutes a day, three times a week. That sounds like a lot. Being physically active is a vital component of pain management because, in addition to all the usual health benefits it offers, for chronic pain sufferers it can also:

- Increase strength
- Increase pain thresholds
- Decrease rebound time
- Encourage and speed healing
- Teach you your body's limits
- Make more routine activities easier
- Encourage healthy sleep
- Release hormones that assist in mental wellness

Starting a new exercise regime can be overwhelming—there is just so much information out there—and adapting an existing one can be scary. What if you make things worse? What if you embarrass yourself? What if you create a new problem?

We are not going to set out any specific exercise routines here; for one thing, it would need to be different for every person. Every single person has to modify their physical activity according to their abilities, their goals, and their time. But knowing your abilities is important, as is setting reasonable goals.

Types of Exercise

Here are some really simple categories of exercise, all of which are recommended for everyone, but in differing ratios depending on your health and abilities.

Stretching

This is always beneficial, and knowing how to stretch properly is very important; it increases mobility, range of motion and flexibility, decreases pain, and softens the impact of more rigorous exercise.

Strengthening

Strengthening exercises are not just about lifting weights; they come in a wide variety of forms, and the simplest often involve using just your own body weight to exercise and tone specific muscles.

Cardiovascular

CV exercise is the type that gets your heart racing and has enormous long-term health benefits. It is often the hardest for those with chronic pain, but, remember, not all CV exercise is equal. There are low-impact options for those who must adjust their practices to their body's needs that will still provide the important benefits you are looking for.

Safe Options for Exercise

There are several types of exercise that are widely considered "the safest" for those seeking to increase their physical activity in the face of existing physical problems:

- Stretching
- Yoga
- Walking

- Pilates

- Strength training

- Aquafit or swimming

And all exercise regimes, regardless of what type they are, should consist of four basic components:

1. Warm-up

2. Exercise

3. Stretch

4. Hydrate

There is almost infinite room within these basic guidelines to create and adapt a variety of possible workouts that will give you all the benefits of exercise without causing harm or triggering your pain disorder.

Know the Difference Between Good Pain and Bad Pain

Exercise hurts. Most of the time, for most people, just a little. You are not really working your muscles or pushing yourself if there isn't some strain, some extra effort that can tire muscles and leave you achy and spent. That's basically why so many people dislike it—it's time-consuming and difficult and do I really have to?!

It's important to know which pains you feel when exercising are *normal* and which are not. Muscle pain, strain or ache is normal after a heavy workout. It means you actually did something, so in many ways this can be considered *good* pain: you tired the muscle out, but that work will make it stronger. Some joint discomfort can also be expected if you have been working on a problem area, but again, this might be a good thing: moving and lubricating problem joints increases their mobility. If you have nerve damage, then this might be triggered by physical strain in the affected area. Normal after-effects such as these should decrease over time and can be temporarily alleviated by icing the area or taking anti-inflammatories.

But remember: no exercise should cause severe pain. Use the pain scale to monitor how you're feeling; if your pain jumps while exercising, stop.

You should not have an increase of more than two points on the pain scale when doing any physical activity.

And none of the following should ever describe what you're experiencing when doing safe exercise:

tweaky	wrenching	acute
burning	yanking	shock
jabbing	ripping	spasming
persistent	tearing	
searing	stabbing	

If you feel anything sudden, sharp, or that isn't alleviated by pausing for a few moments, then stop what you're doing and try something less impactful, smaller, or (if you're having a bad day) simply come back and try again another time, starting slowly and building gradually.

Whatever your situation, your abilities, or your access to resources, there are some simple, common-sense rules you can follow to ensure you are taking the best care of yourself possible in regard to physical activity and pain.

Rules

1. Go at Your Own Pace

You absolutely have to get comfortable ignoring what everyone else is doing. You are not in someone else's body, and they do not know how your body is reacting internally. Whether you're in the gym, in an exercise class, playing team sports, or exercising on your own, you have to be able to read your body's signals and slow down, modify, decrease weight, take a break, or stretch it out, if that is what your body is demanding.

I don't care if the whole room is looking at you; would you rather ignore your body and risk the consequences? Self-consciousness is a natural thing, but it's also a luxury that comes second to pain management. It doesn't matter what the girl in the fancy yoga pants, with her hair perfectly in place, is doing, even if she's running at full sprint without breaking a sweat. Or the muscled, glistening guy in an effortlessly cool cut-off tee with impeccably sculpted muscles. They are not you. It doesn't matter what they can do. If you're nervous about seeming out of place in a class or a team, mention it to the instructor or team captain beforehand. You will establish yourself as forward-thinking, considerate, and someone who is choosing to exercise as best they can *despite* difficult circumstances.

"Hey, just so you know, I have some health issues that might affect my ability to participate exactly as you direct, so if you see me modifying, please don't worry about it."

2. Be Prepared to Consult a Professional

For anyone with chronic pain, consulting a doctor is a smart first step before beginning a new exercise regime. It is—usually—a formality though. Unless you have a very specific problem (e.g. heart-related, blood pressure, lung disease), almost every physician will encourage you to exercise. So let's assume you've done that first step, but now you're standing in the middle of a large and imposing gym with equipment all around you: treadmills and bicycles and bizarre weighted contraptions that somehow must fit a person in there somewhere. You can see what other people around you are doing, but running on the treadmill hurts your knees or affects your balance; the weights are intimidating; the bicycles are all full. What can you realistically do that will improve your physical fitness without causing a pain problem?

This is where assistance—whether online, fitness apps, a trainer, a physio, or even a really knowledgeable friend—can help. It's not about finding the most efficient workout, or how to use every machine, although certainly you can get help with that too. It's about giving yourself a suite of options, so that you have a realistic range of activities that will increase or maintain your fitness level while accounting for whatever you have going on that day. Pain can be extremely limiting, and there is no place where that feels as true as in the gym or when playing a sport. But it does not have to exclude you. You can still exercise if you're having a difficult day, without hurting yourself or making it worse. You just need to know how, what machines you can use when, what your impact and resistance options are, and how to use them correctly.

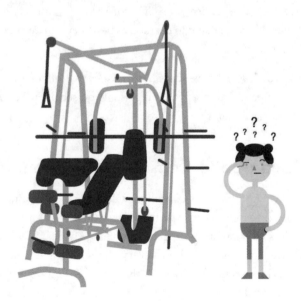

I am constantly astonished by how much difference posture or tiny changes to how you move on a machine can make to your workout. Experts in fitness and body mechanics are valuable resources and ensure you are staying safe and doing impactful work. Do not be afraid to ask people for help; every staff member in the gym should be able to show you how to use a piece of equipment, and you are allowed to ask them to show you at any time. This is what they're there for! Use them!

3. Do Not Medicate to Exercise

If you are in too much pain to do something—anything—then don't do it. That sounds obvious, but when you have a plan, a set *x times a week*, or are part of a team, it can be awfully tempting to push yourself, especially because exercise equals good, right? So it can't be bad to push. But taking pain meds simply to go out and push yourself is self-defeating and is one of those fine lines between reasonable exertion to improve and ignoring your body's feedback. These fine lines are fuzzy, indistinct, and constantly moving, and yes, that's incredibly frustrating. But part of the benefit of exercise is understanding how your body feels in different scenarios and learning the language of your pain. This takes practice.

4. Set Realistic Goals and Monitor Your Progress

Whether you're starting a new exercise routine or continuing with an existing one, constant progress and improvement should be the goal. The rate of your progress is not important. Let me say that again: it does not matter how slowly you improve. If you are working within your body's limits, pushing a little but not hurting yourself, then that is all you can do. Pushing twice as hard will not yield results twice as quickly—in fact, it'll probably set you back. So do not judge your progress, just be mindful of it. When something feels easy, add speed or weight or resistance in small increments. *Small changes are your goal here.* Big changes are risky, difficult to maintain, and unpredictable.

5. Find Something You Enjoy

This may sound impossible, because God knows trying a bunch of different sports and modifying and figuring out which ones you can even realistically do is not a fun chore; in fact, it can drain away all the power that exercise gives you. But, unless you have activities that you can enjoy long-term, pushing yourself to do it will take massive effort, and even more so in the face of existing pain. If you don't enjoy it, you won't do it, period. Find something you can take pleasure in.

Exercise:
Create a Set of
Exercise Possibilities

Try one new form of exercise per month. No, I'm serious. It doesn't have to be anything dramatic—different exercise classes count as something new. A new machine at the gym counts. A new swim stroke. Whatever. Trying something new has great benefits; it can introduce you to a new pleasure; exercise/work a new area of the body; put you in with a new group of people; or inure you to the awkwardness of being the newbie at something. Nothing erodes the luxury of self-consciousness like being the novice repeatedly. And once you are able to stop worrying about what you should be doing, what you look like, and what everyone else is doing, you are free to figure out what actually works for your body. Trying something new and keeping it fresh are key steps toward building a robust, variable, and adaptable set of possible activities you can enjoy.

A note: In any modern gym, every single piece of equipment has a diagram on it with pictures and instructions. These are there for a reason, so use them! Read the details carefully, in particular the guidelines on how you are supposed to sit/stand/transfer your weight. You don't need to pay for a personal trainer if you can't afford one, and you don't have to join a fancy gym. Even basic gyms have staff wandering about or at the front desk whom you can ask for help. Most towns have public pools (usually with aquafit classes), YMCAs with gyms, municipal sports leagues, and a wealth of other options for you. Be creative. It doesn't matter what you do, just that you do it. You can find something you like.

Chapter 5

Boundaries

B oundaries are an integral part of everybody's life, whether they know it or not. They help define who you are, and setting healthy boundaries is crucial for your health and sense of self.

Boundaries are guidelines, rules, or limits that a person creates to identify for themselves what are reasonable, safe and permissible ways for other people to behave around them and how they will respond when someone steps outside those limits. A person can have physical, emotional, mental, sexual, financial, cultural, time, and other boundaries, all of which impact all areas of your life. This is an extensive area of study, particularly in the mental health field, and we're not going to delve into a lot of general information here. For a thorough understanding of boundaries (the what, why, how, when, where, who, and *huh?*), I recommend the Building Better Boundaries study guide by the Self Help Alliance.[4] I actually took this course as part of a group therapy program and found it incredibly educational and helpful for setting my own boundaries, particularly in regard to my health.

Generally speaking, every boundary falls on a spectrum from strong to weak, with healthy boundaries somewhere in the middle, but the two extremes are not so different from one another.

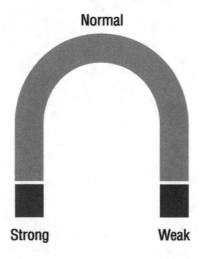

Normal

Strong   **Weak**

---

4   Self Help Alliance, *Building Better Boundaries*.

It is helpful to think of the range of boundary strength as the diagram above depicts; both too-rigid and too-relaxed boundaries can cause physical, emotional, financial, or other problems, but they are closer to each other than you may initially think. The aim is to fall somewhere in the middle—to be able to maintain your sense of self and your own preferences and rights, without shutting people out or losing enjoyment from your life. Having a healthy boundary means you have the strength to say no but allow yourself the option of saying yes. And having healthy boundaries goes both ways: as well as setting your own, you must respect others'.

Healthy boundaries seem like a no-brainer, sort of like exercising, but implementing and maintaining them are hard work. We may allow invasions of our boundaries unthinkingly, through fear of rejection, fear of confrontation, guilt, lack of choice, or safety concerns.

This is true for everyone, but especially so for those living in chronic pain, for whom boundary setting is a vital aspect of self-management. Boundaries can be affected by pain and harder to reinforce when in pain. So, in this chapter, let's look at the major types of boundaries and how they can be affected by your health specifically.

Physical Boundaries

What Is It?

A physical boundary is quite literal—a boundary in space between objects. This may be your personal physical boundary, i.e., your body, or it may be something larger, such as your home, your work space, etc. You have the right to set your own physical boundaries, and this may include rules about when, where, how, and who can enter your personal space.

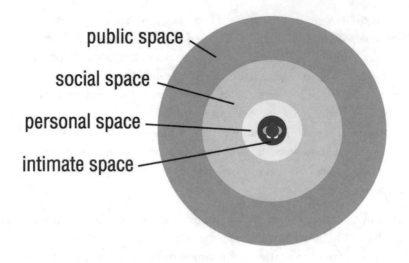

How Does Pain Affect It?

Pain affects physical boundaries in a few ways:

1. Chronic pain sufferers often experience the sensation that their body is not really their own. They have so little control over their experience in it, it can feel like someone else's entirely. This can lead to either porous boundaries ("It doesn't matter what I do, I'm in pain anyway, so why should I care what someone else does?") or very rigid boundaries ("Control is so important, I have to control the manner in which absolutely everything happens to my body"). Pain can make someone shut down their physical boundaries, afraid to let others get close, or it can rob a person of their sense of physical ownership over themselves and lead to a lack of care. Both are dangerous.

2. Another way chronic pain erodes physical boundaries is quite literal—you have to get used to dealing with physical sensations that may not relate to external impetus. Essentially, you may feel physically hurt or weak without an obvious reason. This can play havoc with your sense of physical self, because how can you trust your own body in these circumstances? How can you determine what's right or healthy when logic does not seem to be a factor in how you feel? Again, this can lead to either too-loose or too-strict boundaries, as a reaction to or an attempt to control how you feel.

3. Many chronic pain sufferers have become inured to their personal space and physical bodies being routinely invaded by medical professionals, often for good reason, but, nevertheless, this lack of ability to control when and where and how someone touches you can erode your ability to set boundaries for yourself.

4. Other people may impinge on your physical boundaries by expecting or asking you to do more than you can. These requests may seem reasonable to them—to contribute an equal portion of housework, for example—but the pain you experience makes these tasks harder than they are for other people. Expecting you to be able to do as much physically as a healthy person is a boundary violation, as it ignores what you need to do for your body.

5. And lastly, the simple act of being in pain can affect your physical boundary. You may need physical help which impinges on your boundary. You are probably less able to enforce your boundary because your energies are directed elsewhere. And simply being in pain is a physical invasion that you do not have a choice about. Regardless of all the good work you do elsewhere in setting your physical boundaries, pain will ignore all of it and cut through your boundaries without a second thought. It can be very hard to work on setting your boundaries when you know the monster might burst through the door at any minute and make all your efforts moot.

What Can I Do?

Be clear, be assertive, and be thoughtful. This is true for all boundaries, so let's be specific for the physical:

- Inform someone if you would rather they not touch you or stand too close—do not apologize or feel compelled to explain, just state your preference and do not continue to engage with them until they have respected it.

- It is easier to set your boundaries when you feel well, so make a point of it when you are strong enough to do it, but do not beat yourself up if you're not up to it.

- If your boundary changes with pain, say so, and make sure the people around you know what is appropriate for you in different circumstances.

- If someone routinely ignores your boundaries, tell them so clearly and firmly, and be prepared to move away from them, ask to speak to someone else, leave, or otherwise remove yourself from the situation until you are comfortable.

- If someone close to you requires you to do more than you can, regardless of how you feel, try sitting down and talking to them about their behavior. Many loved ones do not mean to harm us; they are simply being thoughtless about our invisible disease. So educate them about the effect their behavior is having on you.

- Ask to see a doctor or nurse who you have worked with before; if someone new is working on you in an intimate way, introduce yourself and ask them to do the same before starting any procedure. This can remove much of the impersonal aspect of medical interactions.

- Take positive steps to reaffirm ownership of your body; we will look at this in more detail later in the book, but it includes:

  - Seeking out and engaging with positive physical stimuli

  - Exercise and diet, in the sense that they allow you to take more control of your body's intake and output

- Appearance and clothing choices that empower you and reflect your character in a physical, visual way

- Physical self-care without guilt

Emotional Boundaries

What Is It?

An emotional boundary is the ability to distinguish your emotions from others', to separate your feelings from everyone else's. Being able to do this gives you a greater sense of self and grants you permission to feel your own feelings and the ability to choose whether to accept the burden of other people's feelings.

How Does Pain Affect It?

Oof, this is a big one. It is extremely difficult, as a person with chronic health problems, not to feel responsible for other people's inconvenience caused by your illness or pain. When someone has to modify their plans, accept compromises, spend more, accept less, or otherwise change their lives, expectations, or plans because of something inside you—regardless of how little control you have over it—this feels like something you are doing to them, something that you are actively doing but they have no choice in. So, aside from all of the ways this messes with your sense of guilt and expectations for yourself, it also has the effect of putting their emotional reaction on you. Because, if someone gets upset by a change necessitated by your pain, you feel responsible for their upset. You take that on yourself. You feel responsible for making it better.

Whereas, in fact, someone else's reaction to your boundaries has nothing to do with you. At all. They are allowed to be upset or disconcerted or angry by anything—that's their right—but know it has nothing to do with you. Just as your pain is not you, their emotions are not yours. You cannot take ownership of them. This sounds simple, but we all know it isn't, because the natural reaction to expressing a need of our own, when it negatively impacts someone else, is to apologize or back down. But you are not expressing a desire or asking for a luxury—you are expressing a *need*. If someone else can't respect that and has a strong emotional response, that's on them, not you. "Why are you getting angry at me? I am not doing this deliberately."

Another issue with emotional boundaries and chronic pain is that pain can seriously affect mood. You need to have strong emotional boundaries both to protect the people around you from responsibility for your mood, and so that you have the room to feel how you feel. Being in pain is awful and tiring and can make anyone miserable, and you may feel like you have to pretend to be happier than you are, put on a brave face, or somehow get used to it and not experience an emotional reaction. You may feel pressured into allowing someone else to cross your emotional boundary to satisfy their desire to "cheer you up" or otherwise help them deal with their emotional state. Stifling feelings of anger and sadness caused by physical pain is not healthy, but to many it is second nature when dealing with a chronic condition.

It is also extremely normal for loved ones of those in chronic pain to experience guilt, anger, and sadness when they see them in pain. My personal responsibility mantra for this one goes something like: "They are sad because I'm in pain—I am not my pain, but the pain is in me and therefore a function of me—they would not experience sadness if they were not with me—it is my fault because they are with me." This type of cyclical thinking can be brutal, but the truth is, you are not responsible for someone else being sad or angry when you are in pain. That is their response; it may be valid, it may be understandable, it may show they care, but it is not yours. You are not responsible for fixing this for someone else, just as someone else is not responsible for your emotional state.

What Can I Do?

Setting and keeping emotional boundaries requires practice as well as willing participants. If you are a person living with chronic pain, your

family and friends will also need to have their own healthy boundaries
for you to be completely yourself around them. For those that are unable
to do this, you may have to distance yourself from them in times of pain.
There are a few important steps in building emotional boundaries:

1. Recognize that you/the other person is having an
   emotional response.

2. Understand what this response is.

3. Accept this response. Accepting your own emotions is important,
   as is recognizing how another is feeling. This does not mean you
   own their response, just that you see how they feel.

4. Create/find/use strategies that allow you to reduce the intensity
   of this emotional response. This may include asking for time,
   stepping out of the room, having a good cry, etc. In the instance of
   another person's emotional response, you can validate their feelings
   by verbally recognizing them ("I see you are very upset") which
   often helps, or you can, if necessary, reinforce your separateness
   from their emotional response to ensure your own boundary
   is maintained ("You may not continue to yell at me. If you do, I
   will leave").

5. Set small, distracting goals until you are calm enough to deal
   with the issue. For example, many find cleaning to be strangely
   therapeutic. It's also something you probably had to do sometime
   anyway, so it's useful and distracting all at once! By doing
   something else for a while, you are resetting your sense of purpose
   and self, establishing your emotional space from the other person,
   and giving everyone room to process. By keeping your goals small,
   you are ensuring achievability but not allowing anyone time to
   wallow or fester. Perspective is often the most valuable tool in
   accepting your and other peoples' emotional reactions.

Mental Boundaries

What Is It?

Mental boundaries are often very similar to emotional boundaries, but focus more on the way you think and less on the way you feel. Healthy mental boundaries ensure you have your own thoughts, ideas, and opinions without shutting yourself off completely from recognition of or discussion of another person's differing viewpoint.

How Does Pain Affect It?

Chronic pain sufferers are often asked to accept someone else's opinion over their own. Sometimes this is a doctor ("Your experience may be this, but I think you are wrong and should accept my opinion"), sometimes a friend ("I think you can do this, you look fine today"), or a stranger ("You should never take more than three ibuprofen a day, you're over-using"). Always, always, always, your pain comes second to another person's opinion of your pain, unless you exert healthy ownership of your own boundaries.

A slightly more confusing way that mental boundaries are affected by pain is a simple cognitive one: you are less likely to hold strong opinions or be able to think clearly for yourself when in pain or on pain medication. Your intellectual abilities can be massively affected by your physical state, and cognitive impairment is a weak state for mental boundaries.

What Can I Do?

Know yourself, your opinions, and your ideas before engaging another person in conversation about them. Hold on to your opinion if you disagree with them, even if they have letters after their name. If you think a doctor is wrong, say so. If someone is impinging on your boundary or walking over your opinions, say so. If you are in pain and less able to make a clear decision for yourself, say so and ask for more time. Rarely will the decision be urgent and, if you would feel more comfortable waiting until you are sure of yourself, then you have a right to state this. If you have taken medications that are affecting your ability to think and maintain your mental boundaries, remove yourself from the situation or inform the other person what's going on and ask for their understanding and time. Again, this relies on those around you respecting your requests, so learn who does not do this and prepare not to be around them when you are in pain or on meds.

Sexual Boundaries

What Is It?

Sexual boundaries are the boundaries between people with regard to sexual intercourse and all related sexual activities. Healthy sexual boundaries require mutual respect and understanding of limitations and desires between consenting sexual partners.

How Does Pain Affect It?

The desire for intimacy can be severely hampered by pain—both your ability to feel desire and your partner's ability to desire you, whether you are actively in pain or not. Being seen as a sick person is not sexy and can undermine your partner's desire to be with you, even if at that particular moment you feel well ("But you were just projectile vomiting from pain yesterday, I'm so not in the mood"). They may fear hurting you or precipitating an issue they can't control; they may simply be unable to turn off their worry long enough to stoke the necessary impetus to get going. This can be demoralizing and hard to accept for both of you ("What do you mean, you're not attracted to me?!") and should not be ignored or underestimated. And when you are in pain, even if it is mild and you still feel able, your partner may not be willing. This is their boundary and you need to respect it, just as you would expect them to respect yours if you were in too much pain to have sex.

Pain can also affect how you view yourself, your sexual confidence and your belief in yourself as a desirable person. Feeling like a sick person is not sexy either. And of course, pain can cause physical limitations in the bedroom, which again dampens desire and creates the need for modifications and creative thinking.

What Can I Do?

An understanding partner is key here. If you do not feel able to assert your boundaries, especially as they relate to your pain, you will not be able to have a satisfying sexual relationship. It's a sensitive area, but open discussions can greatly facilitate your enjoyment and your partner's. It will also alleviate your and their worry, self-consciousness, and possibility for misunderstandings. It's best to have these conversations apart from amorous activity, as frustration can be high if you have just had a problem or misunderstanding in the bedroom. And remember that Google is your friend—there is almost no sexual problem that someone hasn't encountered before and written about on the internet! Creative thinking and fostering all forms of intimacy—sexual and otherwise—with your partner can greatly expand what's possible and your enjoyment.

Medical Boundaries

What Is It?

A medical boundary is what you are and are not prepared to do, or have done to you, for medical purposes. This includes taking medications, undergoing procedures, and working on therapies, as well as what, when, how, and who can touch you or perform medical procedures. You are the ultimate arbiter of which medical personnel and which medical procedures you are willing to accept.

How Does Pain Affect It?

Choice seems like a faraway thing when living in chronic pain. If you can find someone who may be able to help you or is helping you, fear of losing their help may prevent you from saying no to them. Even if you think something is unnecessary, or will be too painful, you may feel pressure to accept their treatment. We become used to an endless parade of interchangeable nurses and technicians poking us, prodding us, seeing us in flimsy see-through hospital gowns, and accepting their diagnoses and medications unquestioningly. Who has the time and energy to worry about every medical incursion? It's exhausting.

What Can I Do?

Pick your battles. Know for which issues you are willing to accept your doctor's opinion, medications, and prods, and for which ones you need to stand your ground. If you have certain medications which you know haven't worked in the past or have caused unacceptable side effects, or if you know a certain procedure will cause significant pain, be very, very clear about this. State your boundary calmly and ask what alternatives are available. You are the patient—there is very little a doctor can do without your consent! Let your doctor know when and how they may examine you, and if you are not prepared for them to be invasive, say so and work to problem-solve how they can achieve what they need to without crossing your boundaries.

Financial or Material Boundaries

What Is It?

Your financial and material boundaries are about how, when, where, and how much you spend, or use your material possessions—and this being

your decision. You need reasonable control over your own stuff without
undue reference to anyone else.

How Does Pain Affect It?

Others may underestimate or misunderstand your need for an item in
your possession. Friends may ask to borrow your car when you know
you need it to go and pick up dinner ("Can't you just make something
instead?"), ask you to move to a less comfortable chair ("It looks exactly
the same as this one, I don't understand why you're making a fuss"), or
any number of seemingly inconsequential requests and incursions of
your material boundaries. And holding onto your boundaries here can
cause negative emotional reactions from others. It may seem easier just
to lend them what they asked. But you need to use what you need to use,
and you should not have to justify that. You decide how you use your
possessions, and if someone else does not understand that, that is their
weak material boundary.

This is also true of money; being in pain costs a lot. Modifying anything
usually comes with a price, whether it's eating out at a restaurant ("We
can't go there, they only have bar stools and my back won't take it")
or buying a house ("It has to be a bungalow, I can't always manage the
stairs"). This is in addition to the direct cost of medications, therapies,
and treatments—some of which may be doctor-recommended but you
still have to pay out of pocket for.

What Can I Do?

Discuss your financial situation clearly with your doctor when
appropriate. They cannot prescribe you the right meds or the right
treatment if you leave their office and never pursue it because you can't
afford it. Let them know what's reasonable for you, and then work with
them to figure out what's possible within that budget. Generic drugs,
professionals in training, or treatment trials may be available to you,
if you ask.

Be clear about your needs to those around you. If someone asks to borrow something from you, and you don't think you can manage without it (for any reason), then say so. You may feel compelled to explain why, but know that you don't have to. It's yours—you get to do with it what you like.

Setting Boundaries Successfully

Setting boundaries can feel foreign to many of us. Here are some guidelines about how to set healthy boundaries:

- When setting a boundary, do it clearly, calmly, firmly, respectfully, and in as few words as possible.

- Do not justify, get angry, or apologize for the boundary you are setting.

- Have support easily available when you first start setting boundaries. This can be especially useful in the workplace or with family; speak to a sympathetic person first, ensure they know your situation and boundary and what you expect from setting it, and have them present when you set it out to others. Their presence will be comforting, and their response will help guide others.

- You are not responsible for the other person's reaction to the boundary you are setting. You are only responsible for communicating your boundary in a respectful manner. If it upsets them, know it is their problem.

- At first, you will probably feel selfish, guilty, or embarrassed when you set a boundary. Do it anyway and remind yourself you have a right to self-care.

- Always set consequences for those crossing a boundary.

- Follow through on those consequences. Your boundary will be respected if you respect it.

As you might expect, many boundaries overlap, interplay, and affect each other, so figuring out yours can be a complex process requiring a lot of introspection. Remember that it is a learning process—you do not have to be perfect all the time. As you explore and practice setting your healthy boundaries according to or in spite of your pain, you will feel stronger, clearer, and liberated.

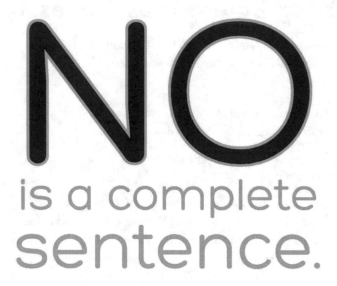

A Note on Saying "No"

Many of us struggle to say no. This is not a function of you but a societal issue, especially for women. Saying no can often seem to mean "I'm not fun" or "I can't" or "I want to be treated differently" or "This is about you" or "I'm disappointing you." It can lead to anger, disbelief, and disappointment, and that's not even counting the effect it has on you and your sense of self. The need to be agreeable or pliable should not trump your pain management (or, frankly, any other part of your life management). Saying no does not mean you are a bad person, are unkind or uncompromising or impolite. We are trained to think that being amiable means always agreeing—it doesn't.

Saying no can feel incredibly hard, especially if you're not used to it, but it's so, so important. Without "no," you can't effectively set your boundaries or take care of yourself. So get used to saying it. Find strategies to make it work for you. You can be considerate, polite, and helpful while still putting your boundaries first.

Exercise:
Identify and Set
Your Boundary

Boundary setting is a massive area of study, and we've really only winged it here as it relates to pain. Everyone is different and your boundaries may change with time, your pain, or who you're with. Here is an easy-to-follow exercise for identifying and setting a new boundary which can be used in any circumstance.

1. Identify the symptoms of your boundary currently being or having been violated or ignored. What drew your attention to the problem? How did you feel during and after the event?

2. Identify the irrational or unhealthy thinking and beliefs by which you allow your boundaries to be ignored or violated. Why did you allow this boundary to be crossed? Were you in danger? Fearful? Too tired? Confused?

3. Identify new, more rational, healthy thinking and beliefs which will encourage you to change your behaviors so that you build healthy boundaries between yourself and others. What are your rights and what are you prepared to stand up for? What do you think you deserve?

4. Identify new behaviors you need to add to your repertoire in order to sustain healthy boundaries between yourself and others. How can you reinforce your rights? In what ways can you protect or distance yourself from habitual boundary offenders? How can you keep your behavior and emotions separate from another's?

5. Implement the healthy boundary-building beliefs and behaviors in your life so that your space, privacy and rights are no longer ignored or violated. Express your boundary clearly, do not justify yourself, and follow through on consequences for boundary-breakers.

Chapter 6

Resource Management

We touched on some of the resources at your disposal in the last chapter—notably financial or material resources, and physical resources—and how you use them, but thinking about all of your resources is a key component of managing your life. This is true for everyone, but especially important for those in chronic pain. How you choose to spend or use your energy, your time, your money, your strength, your emotions, and your body is entirely up to you, and these choices—whether you know it or not—define what is possible for you. If you use all your available energy getting up at six in the morning and spending fourteen hours at work each day, that is a choice, one which leaves you with no energy for hobbies, exercise, friends, family, or self-care. If you choose to spend your time running errands and that leaves you with none to spend with your partner, that is a choice with clear positive and negative consequences.

Resource management is so important for chronic pain sufferers because the emergency store of resources is usually lower for us, and the cushion between plenty and empty is typically much thinner. Essentially, we have fewer physical, emotional, financial, and energetic resources to start with, they run out quicker, and we have less in reserve when we need them. We also bounce back more slowly, so borrowing against tomorrow is harder to deal with. Extra thoughtfulness is required to ensure that you are mindfully and sensibly rationing out what you have available and prioritizing what's important to you.

The spoon theory is a very helpful metaphor that has recently become a popular way to envision the problem we're talking about here. The theory originates from a conversation writer Christine Miserandino was having with a friend one day at a restaurant, where she was trying to explain to her friend how energy management worked for her, a sufferer of lupus. She took a bunch of spoons and explained that each spoon represented the energy needed to complete one task—a normal, everyday task such as making breakfast, having a shower, driving to work, etc. You wake up in the morning and have a set number of spoons, with no way of getting more. This number can vary day by day according to how you feel. Each time you perform any activity, you spend a spoon, and subsequently have less for the rest of the day. You have to consider how many spoons you have in the beginning and ration out what you want to do each day, to ensure you get done what you need to without running out. Christine gave her friend a handful of spoons and then took her through a typical day. For every activity listed, she took away a spoon, until her friend was left with none. What to do then? You have no spoons, no way of getting more, but you still have things to get done, food to make and eat, home to get to—she was stuck!

A lot of healthy people do not have to consider this because they have (seemingly) unlimited spoons, but many with chronic health problems (especially pain, which naturally depletes your spoons faster, as it costs more energy to do the same amount) need to plan. You may already do this without even knowing it, or it might have become a central point in your everyday thinking. Either way, the spoon theory it a helpful way to visualize the issue at hand and can also assist with explaining the problem of limited resources to others. I now have friends who commonly ask me "How many spoons today?"

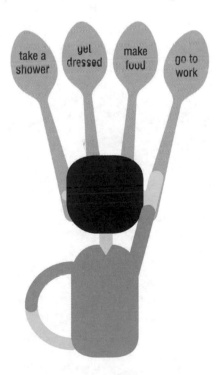

However you choose to ration your own spoons, it is helpful to be
thoughtful about it, to knowingly make decisions about how you spend
your time and energy and everything else. It can take more to do the same
as other people, so ask yourself if something is really what you want to do.

Exercise:
Analyze Your
Resource Spending

We may spend our resources without really thinking. This is particularly true for energy resources; we see others budgeting money, choosing how they spend their time, calorie-counting. But energy management is not normalized in the same way as other types of resources management, because a lot of people don't have to think about it. It's like being the only poor person in a wealthy group of friends going for a night out; only you have to worry about how much the drinks cost. So we fall into bad patterns, and this is counterproductive for pain management and self-care.

The exercise below is designed to help you identify what you might be spending your energy on without knowing it.

1. Choose a typical day—any day, whatever is usual for you.

2. Carry a pen and paper around with you everywhere you go on that day.

3. For every activity you do, write it down and put a check mark next to it. I mean, for *everything* you do. Getting up: one mark. Making breakfast: one mark. Getting dressed: one mark. Doing your hair: one mark. Driving to work: one mark. Sitting in a long meeting: one mark. Walking to lunch: one mark. Going to the store: one mark. And so on for every single thing you do throughout the day, big or small, that spends some of your energy. If you do something particularly strenuous, such as going to the gym, you might even give that two marks.

4. At the end of the day, tally up your numbers. Split your day into
    several major categories (e.g. work, chores, exercise, self-care,
    socializing, hobbies) and work out the total spent in each. How
    much did you spend doing routine chores? How much for work?
    How much for exercise? How much for appearance? How much for
    transport? How much for taking care of someone else? How much
    for preparing or buying food?

5. Now add up the total energy you spent in the day, and for each
    category, divide the category tally by the total. This will give you
    the proportion of your energy that you have spent on each area.
    This is a more helpful number, as it becomes comparable day by
    day, regardless of how much energy you have each day.

6. Compare your numbers. What do they say about your current
    priorities, and is there anything in there that you are not happy
    about? Are you spending 50 percent of your daily energy
    doing chores? Are you spending only 5 percent on hobbies or
    friends? What's eating up your energy, and where do you want to
    spend more?

Example

Monday			
Making Breakfast	1	Driving to Work	1
Eating Breakfast	1	Climbing Stairs	1
Emptying Dishwasher	1	Going Out for Lunch	1
Shower	1	Sitting on Stool	2
Getting Dressed	1	Grocery Shopping	1
Walking Dog	1	...	...

TOTAL: 12

Now split the activities into categories, and sum these. By diving by the day's total, you'll get the proportion of energy spent on each category.

Totals		Proportions	Notes
Work	3	3/12 * 100% = 25%	
Chores	3	25%	
Self-Care	1	8.3%	TOO LOW
Eating	3	25%	
Exercise	2	16.6%	
Hobbies and Socializing	0	0%	TOO LOW
Total:	12		

This exercise can be repeated over various days according to your changing schedule or available energy, to analyze what you're doing by rote and enable you to realign your priorities.

Part 2

MIND AND MOOD

Chapter 7

Concentration and Cognitive Abilities

I n Part 1 we grazed quite a few emotional and psychological factors that can be affected by pain. Here in Part 2, we are going to explore the most significant of these issues individually, so we can better realign our expectation of what is normal and acceptable.

"Hey, I'm temporarily stupider than normal" is not a phrase you ever want to say. It's probably not a phrase you've ever heard anyone say. But it should be. Pain affects cognitive abilities—it just does—and that seems perfectly understandable in the abstract. Making decisions, concentrating, and being rational are all tasks made harder when thinking through a distracting pain, or when operating on limited sleep because of pain. Knowing this and experiencing it, though, are two different things.

Anyone with a chronic pain or neurological disease has almost certainly experienced what is known as "brain fog"—the inability to concentrate, think clearly, or perform usually trivial tasks competently. It can even affect memory. One of the most frustrating aspects of brain fog is that you normally know you're in it; you can see that what needs to be done is achievable and, if you could just focus, if you could just shake yourself clear of it, you'd be fine. On any other day, you know you'd manage, no problem. It doesn't work like that. Knowing you're in the fog does nothing to help you get out of it. The less frustrating but more dangerous version of brain fog comes when you do not realize you are cognitively affected and keep pushing through complex tasks (like driving) when you really shouldn't.

Brain fog is a symptom of many diseases, minor and otherwise, and can present as confusion, forgetfulness, lack of focus, or balance issues. There are many factors that can affect brain fog, including nutrition, exercise, sleep patterns, dehydration, and stress, all of which we can do something about. Sleeping right, eating right, and exercising are all aspects of your greater health care that you are probably doing anyway. But there is no palliative for what may be the main underlying cause of your brain fog: your pain/illness.

However, it's not just an illness itself that can affect your ability to think; medications are notorious for their power to impact your brain function. That might even be their main job (numbing the brain), but taking meds becomes a difficult choice if you know that doing so will diminish your capacity to reason, however temporarily. And for those on constant meds, the continuous background noise of confusion and cotton wool in our minds may have become the new normal, with clarity and competency a distant dream, seen as if through a haze.

There are very few practical ways to avoid pain-related cognitive impairment; if impairment is medication-related, dosing is the most important factor you can control. Taking small amounts at frequent intervals can soften the impact of the drug on your system while still maintaining the necessary levels for your pain management. Exercising, eating well, and drinking plenty of water are the other tools to help avoid general fuzziness. Unfortunately, the only real cure for illness-related fog, though, is rest. Proper rest—staring glassily at a blank wall, empty mind, drooling, taking-a-nap type rest—where you allow your mind to clear, totally, and give it the time it needs to catch up with the rest of your body. Healthy sleeping patterns are essential in health care, and brain fog can be a symptom of tiredness, even when you're getting your eight hours a night. Cognitive rest and time are the only sure-fire solutions to get you back to your normal sharp self.

It is vitally important that you know how to manage yourself and temper the expectations of those around you when you are going through pain-related impairment. Trying to explain what's happening clearly to someone else while you're in pain may well be too much, so ensure your colleagues and family know in advance that you may occasionally and temporarily experience a blip in your normal brilliance. Tell them this in advance so that, when it happens, you don't have to be as eloquent: "Brain fuzzy, words no come" should not be a big surprise to anyone who knows you well. And that's the second part of it—you have to become comfortable admitting it. Yes, this sucks. Yes, we all want to pretend we're Superman and Wonder Woman and always be able to push through everything, and even when our bodies fail us, we're still us! We can still think and remember and be who you know and love! So everything's still alright.

Except we can't, because pain affects that too. It's important to keep in mind this is *temporary* and not a reflection of who you are but is a natural physiological result of what your body is going through. Make sure your friends and family know this too. Mocking you, making fun, pushing you to make decisions, interrupting your mental rest or otherwise invalidating or impinging on your efforts to recuperate while you're unable to think clearly is not acceptable. If you know people who behave this way, find tactics to avoid them when you're feeling foggy. Be proactive; don't wait until you're impaired to try to take action, as this is an inherently flawed method. Sit down when you are thinking clearly and identify what steps you need to take, how you can take them, and who you are comfortable asking for help, then draw up an easy-to-follow action plan for the next time you're in the fog. Simply reacting in the moment is not good enough, as it relies on those about you reacting just as you need them to, without you necessarily being able to tell them what you need.

Shame is a common symptom of cognitive impairment, and the drive to hide it can be overwhelming. You might even be good at hiding it, so those around you genuinely don't know there's a problem. This is not a long-term solution, and it relies on you feeling and feeding a damaging negative emotion. There is nothing shameful about being in pain. There is nothing shameful about having an illness. There is nothing shameful about experiencing a symptom of that illness, and that's all that's going on here. Most people, even annoying ones, will understand and empathize with this when it is explained to them clearly. But shame forces us into half-speech, half-explanations that come out more like "I'm just having a bad day" which, while still true, does not convey the main point. Anyone can be having a bad day, but not everyone has a bad day where they can't reliably make a decision. Minimizing, covering up, and trying to make do are all thoroughly human reactions to potentially embarrassing and difficult personal circumstances, but you have to break that cycle. You have done nothing wrong, so saying "I'm having a brain-fog day, I need you to do this for me" or "Can we wait until tomorrow to decide this, I am having trouble concentrating due to pain"—even if it comes out as, "Can't think, please help"—is allowed. It's what needs to be said in that situation, so own it. Others' embarrassment or confusion is probably a result of your own and is not a reflection upon you.

I may be STUPIDER than normal TODAY, but it'll pass. Your attitude won't.

Chapter 8

Anxiety

Anxiety goes hand in hand with chronic pain; those experiencing long-term health problems are significantly more likely to suffer from chronic anxiety and depression because of the heightened strain their bodies and minds are under. And, as being in pain can cause anxiety, anxiety can exacerbate or even initiate pain. Anxiety can also lower your tolerance for pain. Congratulations! You're screwed in multiple ways!

As two sides of the same coin, a significant part of pain management comes from identifying, understanding, and moving past feelings of anxiousness. Anxiety is so like pain—you cannot solve it, there is no magic answer—but, like pain, it can be unemotionally observed, understood, and ameliorated. You do not have to be a robot to do this, it just takes practice. Knowing what's making you anxious is half the battle in overcoming it, as when you identify the fundamental fears driving your emotions, you can begin to rationally evaluate them. Is this a realistic fear? Is there evidence for this feeling, or am I basing my anxiety solely on my own perceptions? Can I talk to someone about this fear and have an open, honest conversation about its validity? You may not always be able to figure your way out of anxiety, but knowing what's causing it at least gives you the room to choose your responding behaviors. At least be able to choose whether you want to drink yourself into oblivion, rather than doing it without thought.

While there are many ways for anxiety to express itself, there are some common symptoms of anxiety that a chronic pain patient may experience:

- Excessively worrying about physical health
- Trouble sleeping due to worry
- Having nightmares about physical health
- Experiencing panic attacks about prognosis
- Difficulty discussing physical condition
- Avoiding treatments that cause anxiety
- Avoiding social interactions
- Having intrusive thoughts about dying
- Becoming irritable about physical health

Anxiety is not the sole province of those with long-term health problems, but it is more prevalent in us and can make dealing with pain a lot harder. While anyone can feel anxiety at any time and for almost any reason, there are some common triggers for chronic pain sufferers that underpin most pain-related anxiety.

Are Any of These Familiar?

 I can't do this. I'll fail, be humiliated, show my weakness.

I have to hide how sick I feel.

I might not be able to do this in the future. My pain is unpredictable, so I have to take every advantage now and not stop, because any day, the tide might turn and I'll be stuck, unable to do what I want.

This feels worse than normal; what if something new has come up? What if I'm getting sicker?

What if this makes me worse? I don't have the capacity to deal with more, my partner doesn't have room for anything else to go wrong. I'd be safer not trying. I can't take any risks.

I can't cope with this. I am not capable, it's too much, I am overwhelmed.

How do I make the right decision? The outcome may be serious and/or unsalvageable; what if I make a mistake?

There are so many compromises, so many difficult decisions to make, how do I know which is the best? I am overwhelmed having to constantly make these decisions/choices/compromises.

I can't take care of myself and get everything I need done. There's too much, something's going to give.

What if that other person doesn't believe me? My pain is invisible; what if I can't properly convey the way I feel? What if the doctor thinks I'm making it up? How will I get help?

Is it all in my head? How do I know I'm not doing this to myself? What if this isn't an understandable medical issue, but a figment of my own brokenness?

What if that person decides this is too much to deal with and leaves me? How will I manage on my own? How will I ever find someone willing to put up with doctors and medical crises and compromises? How can I bear disappointing my partner again?

What if I can't take care of my kids/parents/family? I am failing as a parent, as a spouse, I can't engage the way I want to, I can't join in and share the fun, I might as well not be here.

What if what's possible for me is not enough? How will I live with these continuing compromises? How will my partner accept them? What if this isn't enough for me?

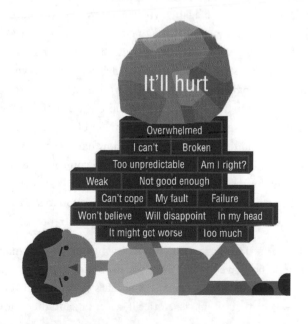

Unpredictability seems to be the foundation of many of these worries, and unfortunately it is one of the most difficult aspects of chronic pain to overcome. How you change, your prognosis, your treatment, and your own and your family's ability to cope can and probably will morph over time; this is just another thing you cannot control. We know we're not gods, but at this point most of us have to accept that, at times, we barely have more control over ourselves than babies.

Acceptance is the only real path to moving forward, past these issues and the difficulties of what may happen in the future; you don't know what's going to happen. No one does. You can't predict how something is going to make you feel. You can't know what's going on in someone else's head or how well they are coping—and even if you could, would it help? All you can do, every day, is accept what you have in front of you and make the best-informed decisions you can. Yes, that's a pretty dull answer, and Christ it can be boring and a lot of hard work. Way too much hard work. Why do you have to do all this hard work just to exist when other people don't have to? Drinking to oblivion without having to think about it may seem like an attractive alternative. Fun? Yes. Healthy? No.

It's important to acknowledge success. Success is not measured against a healthy person's abilities, but against your own. If you have improved in some way—through treatments, through efforts on your own, through support—in really any field related to your health and your ability to manage, then this is a success. You need to celebrate your growing ability to live with chronic pain. Every time you don't drown your sorrows and anxieties but choose to face them—that's a success. It is not an easy thing to do; so many of us use the unrealistic barometer of an ideal, healthy person and so, no matter how well we do or how hard we try, we always seem to fall short. Be kinder to yourself—observe your own behavior and note when something has changed for the better. It will empower you, give you back a small measure of control, and allow you to see the bigger picture of your health rather than staying stuck in the trenches.

You need to get used to "I'm anxious about my health" as a normal part of your life; you do not have to justify it, there does not need to have been a change to instigate the worry. It just is. And that's okay. You don't have to make it go away or fix it. It just is. Notice it, accept it, and then move on.

Chapter 9

Anger

Frustration. Yep, that's pretty understandable. Being angry at life, God, yourself, friends, family, everyone—there's plenty of anger to go around. No need to ration it, there's enough for everyone. Anger at your health, your situation, your pain, your body, other people's health, other people's inability to understand, other people's kindness or concern or worry or attempts to help, other people's thoughtlessness, misdiagnoses, diagnoses, your doctors, your own expectations, your own failures…the list is potentially endless. Everything, good or bad, can make you angry when you are living inside a body that experiences chronic pain. Just because it's natural, though, does not mean you can indulge in it.

Research shows that anger, like anxiety, can actually worsen pain. Anger:

- Increases pain intensity

- Decreases pain tolerance

- Negatively affects sleep

- Promotes unhealthy coping behaviors which can also affect your pain

- Causes friction with caregivers

So yeah, it's bad. Anger increases heart rate and breathing rate, releases adrenaline, tenses muscles, and heightens awareness. None of which help you feel better.

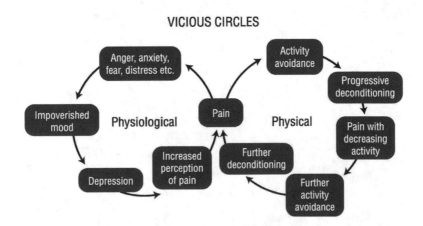

VICIOUS CIRCLES

Anger can have a useful purpose: signaling to you that something is wrong and giving you the fuel to fight or change it. Anger about a health condition, however, is a sensitive topic. It's common to hear of cancer survivors who "fought" cancer, who "battled" or "beat" or some other aggressive verb that depicts their heroic struggle against an invading force in their body. You don't hear much about chronic pain survivors; the struggle is no less epic, no less significant, but can't be thought of as a battle. There is not something to be won—the very definition of a chronic problem is that there is no solution, it is perpetual. There's no glory in a never-ending, slow, plodding resistance to pain. I can't help but give a bitter laugh when I hear the term "survivor" for someone who has experienced what may well have been a devastating but ultimately temporary illness. They get to get better, to return to normal. Yes, the threat of death might have been there. But it was a binary choice, black or white. Get better or die. Stark, but simple.

Pain is about living in the gray areas. There is no definitive better or worse—most chronic pain sufferers are unlikely to die directly because of their chronic pain disease. Anger at other people's options and perceived heroism is just one aspect of the anger your own chronic pain causes. Being angry at a temporary medical condition may well be a useful tool, giving you the energy and strength to fight and win, but anger at a long-term, chronic illness is only counterproductive, wasted energy that harms your body and mind. Short-term anger may be a tonic, but long-term anger is a toxin. It will harm you if not managed. And managed does not mean repressed; there is a growing amount of scientific evidence that suggests inhibiting anger can be as bad for you as indulging in it, heightening pain diseases such as fibromyalgia. So you can't ignore it either.

There is a wealth of information available for those experiencing significant anger issues, with special counselling, support groups, and even medications available. Most of us know what anger looks like in short bursts: yelling, reddening, gritting teeth, aggressive behavior, feeling resentful and sick. It's important to recognize how your own anger manifests and to cultivate strategies to break the negative cycle. Negative thoughts lead to a physical response, which causes pain, which leads to more negative thoughts. We need to add a step between thoughts and the physical response so as to not inflame or aggravate our physical conditions.

Here are a few simple tips for recognizing your anger before it leads to a physical response or action:

1. Be aware of your environment. There may be triggers that always cause anger; identify and avoid them.

2. Be aware of physical changes in your own body. Know if your heart begins to race, your palms become sweaty, you tense up. These are all warnings signs of anger.

3. Be aware of your behavioral changes. It may be pacing, yelling, impatience, sarcasm—but notice if you begin to act differently.

Once you have identified that you are angry, you need to find a way to calm down before you explode. Some suggestions:

- Deep breathing

- Count to ten before reacting

- Muscle relaxation techniques

- Meditation

- Cognitive awareness—be aware of how your actions are affecting your loved ones and others around you

- Find something to defuse the situation

- Redirect your thoughts to something else

Now that you have a handle on your anger, you could choose to bury it, but a far healthier alternative is to find a way to channel it, thereby addressing the fundamental emotion without letting it control you. Again, this is nowhere near as much fun as letting loose, screaming, saying *fuck it* to all the sensible efforts to take care of yourself and everyone else and just being. Just being angry can sometimes feel really, really cathartic. But, again, it's not in the best interests of your long-term health.

So try to find assertive rather than aggressive responses—stand up for yourself and your needs; be firm without being angry. Understand that anger is usually a secondary emotion and, instead of letting it control all of your focus, identify and problem-solve the underlying cause. And don't forget that other people have needs you may not be aware of. Do not assume you are the only person dealing with a need; take time to consider another person's need before reacting.

You have a right to be angry; anger is valid, and it doesn't have to be finite. Even the kindest, humblest, and most reasonable person will occasionally, or even often, become very angry at chronic pain and all of its effects. Putting your best foot forward is pretty tough when both feet hurt. The anger, though, just like the pain, is no one's *fault*. You can't blame anyone, yourself included. So you can let it affect you, define your behavior and thoughts and in some ways your physical health, or you can choose to redirect that energy elsewhere. That decision is entirely yours.

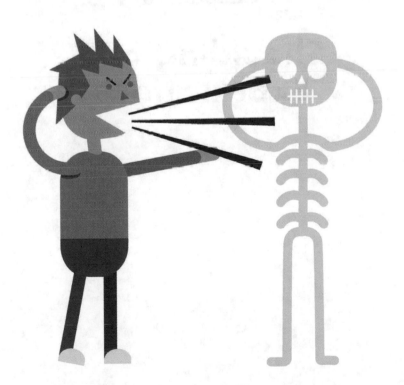

Chapter 10

Shoulding and Expectations

Are you shoulding all over yourself? This is one of the best questions I have ever been asked, and it has stuck in my head because of its aptness. Shoulding is something we all (except the most virulent narcissists) do, whether we know it or not, and it can seriously affect our mood and our health. "I should have done this, I should be able to do that, I should manage this, I should know what to do, I shouldn't have asked for help, I should be able to do this without meds, I should I should I should." Should defines us, our expectations for ourselves and for others. We don't just do it to ourselves: "He should have known better." It's how we measure what we think is possible, how we want to act and think, and how we want others to act and think. But all too often, shoulds are not realistic, and they always have the benefit of hindsight.

The chronically-in-pain have a lot of really specific shoulds. "I should be able to do this. I shouldn't be drawing attention to myself. I shouldn't ask for help. I should have stayed at home. I should have done something easier. I should have made it harder. I should be better by now"—all of which rely on one fundamental, flawed assumption: that there is some measure, some yardstick against which you and your behavior and your pain are being held and judged. That someone, somewhere, themselves utterly perfect and never failing to do or say exactly the right thing, has this yardstick and is doing the judging. Leaving religion aside—because, frankly, if your particular god is judging you for your ability to deal with pain, then I don't really want anything to do with him/her/it/them—this is patently untrue. But what about family? What about colleagues and bosses and strangers? Well, yes, some of these people may be judging you. Welcome to the human experience. But none of these people are perfect, none have the ideal yardstick of how someone in exactly your position should feel or behave or think, and none of them are experiencing what you are experiencing. You are the only person who has to carry your pain. There is no one right answer on how to deal with any given problem, how best to cope, how to react in every situation. There is simply a range of possibilities, some better than others, any of which may or may not work. What's right today may not be right tomorrow.

Even the most judgmental, harshest of these people are busy dealing with their own lives and their own problems, and shoulding all over themselves as well. There is not a human alive that doesn't have some problem, health, relationship, career or otherwise, that they are dealing with at any given moment, and the assumption that they have time to concentrate only on you, analyze you and your behavior and make accurate, justifiable observations is an enormously self-centered delusion, one that we all share. Just as you worry that they are judging you, they worry that you are judging them. So give yourself a break, as you would to a friend. Everyone is the center of their own world and it's understandable to think that your behavior, particularly as it relates to something as important and pressing as your pain, is easily discernible and a high priority to those around you. It's not. Their pain is the center of their universe, and this is true even if you're happily married, even if you have kids, even if you have the best, most supportive people in your life. It's human nature. So a little perspective, knowing that you are the only person who truly has the right to should yourself, is the first step in freeing yourself from unrealistic expectations. The second step is catching yourself in your shoulds and figuring out where they come from—are they valid, and are they really helping?

There may be some people in your life that don't care or don't believe your pain, who should you in specific and targeted ways. We'd like to think those who care about us wouldn't do this, but experience begs to differ. "You should do more" or some variation on that complaint is a fairly standard attack for chronic pain sufferers. It's hurtful, shaming, and thoughtless, and it makes us want to do more, do better, be better. Or to argue, prove somehow that our experience is valid. There is no quick fix for dealing with people who refuse to honor your personal experience, and walking away is often the only way to avoid a more serious breach. Remember: you do not have to accept the premise of their statement. They are speaking based on flawed assumptions; it is not your job to constantly correct them, and it is not your job to make them feel better. They are living in a different version of reality—don't get sucked into it.

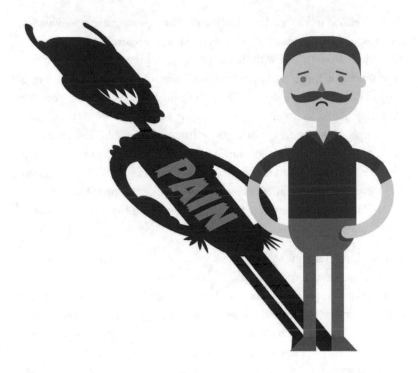

Expectations for chronic pain sufferers are tricky things, partly because the goal posts seem to be constantly moving, and partly because they reinforce your otherness. Other people may have similar expectations—the able-bodied may, for example, expect to be able to walk up a hill without effort. Physical expectations, especially based on appearance, are very common socially, and it can be devastating when you fail to meet them. It doesn't matter if they were unreasonable expectations; it still feels like failure. Expectations of symptoms based on illness are also common; when your personal experience deviates from a perceived norm, when you do not match someone else's anticipation of an illness or its related symptoms, or your ability to deal with these symptoms, this can create tension and lead you, the actual sufferer of the disease, to second-guess yourself. You hold yourself up to standards based, not on your experience or how you are feeling, but on someone else's—often second- or third-hand—opinions.

Complications from well-known ailments can be easily dismissed as inconsequential or passed over as normal and therefore unimportant. The elderly have to deal with this all the time—"Of course you are experiencing arthritis pain, you're eighty." Age or expectation that it might happen doesn't mean it doesn't hurt. The pain is just as real as if you were a thirty-year-old feeling it. Dismissing your pain as expected is callous and simply allows others to move on without feeling obligated to worry or care. This also happens to women experiencing dysmenorrhea (severe menstrual cramps). Pain is expected, is perceived as routine, and therefore those experiencing heightened pain are more likely to be subjected to others' false expectations of how they should be dealing with it. "It's only period pain, everyone has it, stop whining."

You need to filter your world. Just as we remove bad people, bad food, or bad experiences from our day-to-day, you need to remove bad expectations. Surround yourself with realistic expectations for yourself and your family, and ensure those around you have similar expectations—it can avoid a lot of unnecessary heartache. It will also give you a better understanding of your pain, your boundaries, and your abilities, as you stop trying to do what you think you should be doing and start focusing on what your body is actually telling you.

You may discover that a lot of your shoulds are in fact "I want to be able tos," which is both understandable and a lot less loaded. A lot of people have "I want tos" without achieving those goals, and that's just part of life. Consider which of your shoulds are in fact wants (for yourself), and which are shoulds (for other people).

Feel Free to Be Weird

Don't be afraid to get weird. Genuinely, one of the most valuable changes in my own self-care has come from ceasing to give a shit what other people think—what other people's shoulds are. So, okay, I carry my own cushion into the cinema. That may get me looks, but I'd rather be comfortable. I will request a certain type of chair at a restaurant, and stand and politely wait as the wait staff, and finally manager, run about trying to fulfill my request. Some may think I'm being difficult, but I know I'm taking care of my back. Dinner out does not have to mean immobility tomorrow. If you need to sleep with props—wedges and pillows and whatnot—then do so. No one else can get your sleep for you. Buying clothes can be a tough one—nothing is ever made for modification, so getting creative is a necessity if you have specific physical restrictions. Practice will teach you that most people will make a genuine effort to help you, without you having to explain yourself or apologize. So if you need to wear maternity clothes and you're a twenty-year-old guy, go for it. Walk into the maternity store and ask for the help you need. You don't know those people, who cares what they think? If you need to carry your own suite of cushions, blankets, props, meds, and heat pads wherever you go, then do. You do not have to ask anyone's permission; you are free to take care of yourself however you see fit. No one is keeping score, tracking your changing needs or weirdnesses. No one cares, not really. So what's stopping you?

Chapter 11

Consistency, Goals, and Giving Up

Consistency is great. Knowing what to expect is almost always the preferred option, unless you like surprises, and even then I'm willing to bet you only like the good ones. "Surprise" and "health" are not really two words you want in the same sentence. That's what we have to deal with, though, because chronic pain is very often the same thing as chronic inconsistency. You don't know what your body is going to do when you wake up in the morning; is it going to be a good day? Or are you going to wake up and be in pain? Will your back seize up today, or will you be able to get everything done? A lovely lurking surprise at the end of your bed; you know it's going to be there when you wake up, it haunts you as you go to sleep. Some people have chronic pain that is absolutely, depressingly predictable—if I do this, I will hurt—but for most of us there is an element of randomness in our bodies that we simply can't ignore.

It sucks. Consistency is a wonderful thing, having something reliable, something predictable, even if it's a bad something, can often feel better than the not-knowing of inconsistency. Chronic pain does this to us—it takes away normal because how can there be a normal when there is no standard? So go ahead, you can say it. It's shit. This is shitty. It's an all-out fuckfest of humiliating, draining, exhausting, confusing, and infuriating incomprehensibility. Inconsistency and unpredictability are possibly the worst aspects of living with a chronic pain problem, and a lot of negative psychological effects are rooted in them. You cannot trust your body, and this is one of the most frightening realizations a person can have.

It doesn't just impact you. You become the inconsistent person; your loved ones and coworkers have to deal with this too, and some can't. Some simply cannot cope with the randomness, and I find it hard to blame these people because I know that if I had a choice, I'm not sure I would choose to deal with it either.

PAIN LIES

For those of us enjoying a chronic disease, we have no choice. So what to do? I ache for consistency, for the ability to get out of bed every morning and know I can reliably perform a range of tasks without the need to lie down, take meds, faint, cry, or otherwise react negatively. I yearn for my partner to be able to rely on me, to be able to make plans and know we can keep them, and not always have a back-up plan or exit strategy in mind, just in case. Consistency is a laudable goal, but it may not be an achievable one. For those just beginning to understand their physical limitations, it will take some time to establish a reasonable set of boundaries. These boundaries are usually found through trial and error and can be more quickly unearthed through systematic testing and rigorous documentation. So, for example, if you want to cook a certain meal, perform a certain chore, do a certain exercise—anything, really— then do it, and record how you feel. Did it negatively impact your pain in any way? Try it another day, and again, write down how you feel. If there's a lot going on and you're not sure which activity is prompting which reaction, take a quiet day and stress-test yourself. Do just one thing and see how you feel. If one particular activity is consistently harder or causes more pain than you are prepared to accept, note this. Avoid it. Or, if you cannot avoid it, schedule it on days where you have fewer other commitments. Do this with everything, large and small.

At first it seems like a lot of effort, but it will become second nature and soon you will have a good understanding of what is possible for you on any given day, depending on how you feel. Absolute consistency is not possible, but a reasonably certain range of consistency is. Find the spread between doing nothing/feeling well and doing everything/feeling awful, and work around the middle point between the two. Start small—small deviations around what you think is possible to test how you feel—and, with time and practice, you will get better at monitoring yourself and managing your pain levels. Bigger changes won't become quite as definitional as they have been. You will start to be able to manage more without throwing yourself for a loop. Consistency becomes more likely, even if it can't be promised.

An Aside on Goal-Setting

Setting goals for ourselves is a major tool in managing our health. Whether it's a food goal, a meds goal, an exercise goal, a weight goal, a personal time goal, a family goal, or a career goal, wanting to improve our lives is part of the human condition. This gets a little harder when health throws obstacles in our way; suddenly our energies are focused on the health issue or pain rather than the goal, and, before you know it, time has passed and you've missed an opportunity or a deadline or simply regressed. Achieving goals while physically ill requires determination. It's not enough to set a goal and work toward it. You have to be realistic from the outset, knowing that unexpected issues may complicate the matter; you have to constantly adapt to how your health is affecting you, affecting your priorities and energy levels; you must be prepared to reevaluate your goal and accept changes or compromises you might not like. Modifying your goal is not a sign of failure; it is a step in the collection of better data and will eventually get you to where you want to be. This is not an impossible task, but it requires time and effort.

Many sufferers of chronic pain feel stuck in their lives and their situation, as if their pain is dictating all aspects of their lives. Their horizons have been artificially narrowed, and they don't know what to do about it. You absolutely can affect material change in your life, but you have to accept that it will be hard. Breaking down goals into small, achievable, and recognizable steps is a very helpful method to work toward your goals in a healthy way. Analyzing everything minutely may be frustrating—you may experience a strong sense of *I just want to do it already*—but even this can be helpful in identifying what's really important to you. If it's not worth the work, why are you doing it?

Knowing when to stop and when to push is another issue that comes up a lot when making changes; pushing too hard toward a goal might get you there sooner, but it might cost a lot in terms of your pain. Stopping feels like failure but may be required for a short period of time to give your body the space it needs. If you find yourself having to stop, re-examine what you're doing. Maybe you can break the change into smaller steps, so your body does not react as strongly. Pacing yourself is a massive task for anyone with chronic pain and can become one of those pesky inconsistencies we talked about earlier: some days you can push, some days you have to stop. Stopping and starting when working toward a goal is not stopping and starting your dedication to the goal; it's just a pause as your body catches up. Don't dramatize it. Pausing is healthy, and proactive pausing is better for you and your goal in the long run than pushing full steam ahead and then crashing.

Giving Up Is Healthy

Giving up gets a bad rap. Quitter, dropout, shirker, slacker, failure, loser, deserter—no one wants to be this. No one wants to say something, then not do it, or make a promise and fail to deliver, or set a goal and not meet it. Letting go is a big part of everyone's life and an even bigger part of a chronically-in-pain person's life. You have to let go of so much, including the image of yourself as Superman. This can be galling, gutting even. It is, however, a fact of life and one you will have to accept. You cannot do everything. You cannot achieve every goal you set for yourself. Even the carefully planned, well-thought-out, and reasonable goals may sometimes be unachievable. There are times when you have to choose to walk away. Pushing through no matter the consequences, ignoring your body's physical reactions, is not a sensible alternative to giving up. Yes, you might care about this goal or this promise. Yes, it might cause you significant heartache to let it go. But giving up versus hurting yourself? In 99 percent of cases, hurting yourself is an extreme and unnecessary response.

Giving up gracefully is another matter entirely. Letting go of your goal and letting go of kicking yourself for it are two different things, and just as you have to learn when to give up, you have to know that it's okay to give up. Reasonable—better, even. Walking away can be a mature, reasonable response to a situation or even a person, but convincing yourself of this is probably harder than the actual walking away.

Spontaneity

The flip side of the consistency problem is spontaneity. Our bodies need consistency, and we naturally aim for this in the face of all the unpredictability we experience, but doing so rules out a pretty important aspect of fun: spontaneity. There is no jumping into a car for an impromptu road trip when you have to prepare and plan everything beforehand. There are no unthinking decisions just for the hell of it, because the stakes are too high. The young and unburdened, especially, rely on spontaneity and the freedom to do whatever they like because it is their right, one experienced and expected without thought. When you can't do this, young or old, and those around you can, it's extremely demoralizing. You lack a fundamental freedom—the freedom from having to worry about your body. You physically need the boredom of day-to-day consistency and that boredom is, well, pretty damn boring. Aiming for boring is a lousy endeavor. Watching others change plans, carefree, at the drop of a hat, do whatever they please without apparent concern, is defeating. Even if you do everything right, take amazing care of yourself, strive for your best life, you will probably never reach the stage where spontaneity is a viable option.

This is one of the seemingly small but inescapable facets of chronic pain, perhaps trivial in itself but that adds to the weight of not-normal that grinds you down day after day. And accepting that as part of your life will be, like so many acceptances, an ongoing struggle, and one that will only disappear with your pain.

Chapter 12

Strength Euphoria and Setbacks

Here's an important note on strength euphoria. You might have a different name for it, but you know the feeling: the one that comes when suddenly, maybe because of extra work you've been putting in, maybe due to a new treatment, or maybe for no reason at all, you feel stronger. Better, more capable. Activities that caused serious pain in the recent past are now manageable; when you push, it delivers results rather than setbacks. This is a wonderful, surprising feeling, but don't let it go to your head. Jumps forward are as unpredictable and as undependable as setbacks. Feeling better or stronger is great, and if you are able to do more, then do more. But beware of the easy trap: "I feel good, I feel well, I am better. I can do anything." Suddenly you are Wonder Woman again, and it's all the more wonderful because of the relief from pain. Staying level and calm during these times is trying but necessary. In order for the improvement to even have a chance of being more than temporary, continuing to pace yourself and monitoring your pain is essential.

If you're prepared for strength to come and go at random, to just let it be and take full advantage of it when it arrives without concern for long-term improvement, that is a perfectly valid choice, but it does come with a greater emotional tax. You have to be fully prepared, when and if things deteriorate, not to blame yourself or what-if all over yourself. If you can do this, then great, have at it. The smoother, less taxing option is to gratefully accept any improvement, but not pin all of your hopes on it. You might be better permanently. It might be a small movement in a generally upward-trending curve. It might be a reprieve before a worsening. The point is, you can't know. Only time will tell. A Zen attitude of acceptance is important so as to not upset your self-management progress or begin to ignore re-emerging signs of chronic pain. The euphoria from feeling better, even partially, can be overwhelming, so just be mindful of how you let it affect your continuing pain management efforts.

A similar point must be made for setbacks. Setbacks are hard to accept and, in the moment, can feel like absolute failure. Something got worse— it's the end of the world. It takes perspective and practice to come to see these as minor data points in a much larger, more complex picture of your health. It might be the start of a worsening, it might be a reaction to something temporary, it might be nothing at all. Again, only time will tell, so don't let it define your mood or your management strategies. Only when a change persists should you, calmly and with your doctor and family, choose to reevaluate your ongoing plans.

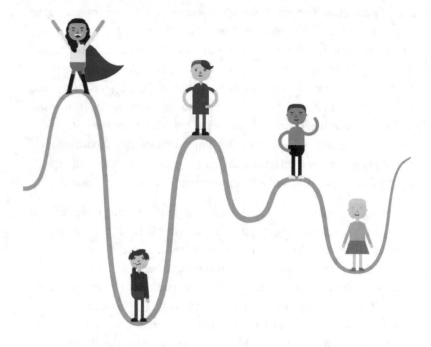

You will also—absolutely—experience setbacks in your own pain management. You will struggle to put yourself first, to be calm in the face of pain, to make smart choices every time. Nobody is perfect, and nothing discussed in this book is easy. Sometimes you're going to feel better, sometimes worse. Sometimes you're going to do really well, and at other times you won't be able to cope. The practice of pain management is a long-term one, a lesson to be constantly learned. Every day is different, and each new day is a fresh challenge in how to manage your pain and your life.

Chapter 13

Career

Your career is probably an important part of your life. Many of us define who we are—at least in part—through what we do for a living. Being good at something gives us self-confidence and empowers us. Doing work you enjoy is a privilege, one that not everyone has. And working toward career goals, even if it's not in your dream career, is a big aspect of how you and others measure achievement. Living with pain can seriously affect your ability to apply yourself to a career, dedicate your energies and time, advance as you wish, or, in some cases, work at all and earn the money you need to live. Ill-health, especially when young, materially disadvantages us in the workplace. This is not a minor side effect or an ignorable consequence. Work is vital to most of us. Money is vital to basically all of us. The ability to support ourselves and our families, contribute to a workplace, and live up to our own expectations are powerful drives. The inability to do these things can be a direct cause of depression and feelings of inadequacy and helplessness.

Let's not mince words. Living with pain will probably prevent you from starting certain career paths. Want to be an ER doc? Can you stay on your feet for twelve to fourteen hours at a time, skipping meals and feeling no ill effects when you do so multiple days in a row? No? Then you're not going to be an ER doc, and if you know you have a chronic pain condition when you're eighteen, that's a quick decision. And sometimes it is that simple. Often it's not. Many workplaces and jobs have more complex requirements that may mean some physically strenuous activity, but not all the time, and are potentially modifiable. For those young enough to still be considering the best career route, knowing your limitations from the get-go is everything. Be realistic about what you can and can't achieve. Be realistic about what you can expect from your chronic pain and if there is even the chance it'll ever improve. This may be demoralizing and gut-wrenching, to consider what you want to do with your life and then maybe have to accept that you can't, but it is better to do that from the outset than waste precious time and energy chasing a pipe dream. You are in your body for the rest of your life, and the decisions you make today about what to do with it will stay with you forever.

For many, chronic pain only becomes an issue once a career path is already begun. Your pain may be due to a lingering injury or it may herald the start of a long-term disease. You may be settled permanently somewhere; you may be in a workplace that can meet your new needs, or you may not be. This heavily depends on what you do, how old you are when your pain becomes an issue, and what you can expect from your pain. The older a worker is, the easier it is to modify and adapt existing job requirements to meet your new abilities. It's also more likely that you will have coworkers of similar age doing a similar thing. A lot of workplaces with older staff already adapt to meet special requirements and see no problem doing so. Smaller businesses and physically driven businesses are the exception here, and if you work in either and suddenly find yourself needing to change how you work, or even how much you work, being up-front with your boss is vital. The majority of people, when approached openly and with genuine intent to problem-solve, will not ignore your requests to discuss and brainstorm ways for you to stay employed with them. Those who do ignore employee health issues can expect 1) lawsuits, and 2) a high employee turnover.

If you find yourself needing to modify your work because of chronic pain, you need to know where you are in terms of your body. What is no longer possible? What can be done instead? Are there simple solutions your employer could support that will make your work possible or easier? Think before you speak; have a comprehensive list of concerns and possible solutions ready, then speak to your boss. No, it may not be perfect, but you will probably be able to figure something out to ensure you can still work in some capacity.

All of this relies on reasonable people taking you at your (or your doctor's) word and being willing to accommodate you. This is not guaranteed, and you should be prepared for some people, colleagues and bosses, to be unwilling to adapt or change to fit your needs. If you have been reasonable, explained the situation, and still get no traction, then you know to move on. Investing energy and time into lost causes is not a luxury you have. Some naysayers can be ignored totally without impacting your work product, but if a colleague or boss is preventing you from being able to do your work by being inflexible, then have an escape plan. Know when to cut your losses and move on, and be sure when talking to new potential employers that you emphasize your previous

work's unwillingness to accommodate reasonable medical requirements
as a reason for leaving. Be the one who terminated the relationship—that
way you are someone who looked after yourself and was reasonable, not
someone who was fired for mysterious medical reasons (which may be an
employer turnoff).

On top of all this is the potential that you can't work at all and need to
live on disability, short-term or long-term. Your options here depend
enormously on where you live, your health benefits, and whether you
have a doctor in your corner—as every disability benefit option will
require sign-off from a medical professional. The decision to apply for
disability is a huge one, and, for many chronic pain sufferers, it's one that
gets put off repeatedly. You really want to be able to work and the thought
of stopping, for any period of time, feels like an admission of failure.
What if you can't ever work again? There's a holiday coming up, or there's
concern about the loss of work-related health benefits. Wouldn't it be
better to push through, or to wait for a better time?

Unfortunately, there is no such thing as a good time to go on disability,
and the decision to do so is a deeply personal one. Talk with your doctor
if you are struggling to work and do so proactively. Some disability benefit
claims take a long time to process, so forethought and planning are always
helpful, if at all possible. Part-time or freelance work is a great option for
those with ongoing health issues, as this allows you the option to work
your own hours and to earn some income, without the stresses, schedule,
and demands of a full-time job.

All of this may sound very practical in theory but can be heart-rending
or simply not an option in actuality. Saying goodbye to the dream of a
particular career or a long-held job are very difficult decisions, not to be
taken lightly. Just another fun example of feeling *less than*. And many are
struggling just to get by, and the almighty decision to leave a well-paying
job is too big to comprehend. The truth is you may not have that choice
right now—but know your options and start having a strategy in mind.

Do not be fooled—none of the above is intended to make this process
sound easy. It just contends that hefty doses of assertiveness, self-care,
and realism factor into your planning. Have a good support network in

place, both at work and at home, to help you deal with the consequences of your changing health on your career. It may well become important for you to find other sources of self-confidence and esteem outside of work, to ensure you still feel useful and capable even if you cannot work as you wish. Volunteering is a great resource for this, as many volunteer organizations are designed to allow people with varying abilities to participate and provide you with an outlet to be genuinely useful to others. Hobbies are also great tools for separating your sense of self from the workplace.

Realism is a hard pill to swallow, and the urge to think of chronic pain problems as temporary and therefore not requiring major lifestyle changes can be intoxicating. Don't fool yourself. Being realistic about what you can and cannot do, and accepting that, is the first step toward finding a career path that will fulfill your intellectual, aspirational, or financial desires without compromising your health. You can find a solution that will work for you, not just who you want to be, but your physical body as well. But you're in your body, whether you like it or not, so you better get used to it, or you'll find yourself down a path that's very difficult to change.

Chapter 14

Relationships

Relationships are hard even in the best of circumstances; adding in ill-health, pain, unpredictability, and uncertainty makes the need for honesty, communication, and personal responsibility crucial. There are a wide variety of people in your life who will be affected, to some degree, by your chronic pain condition. Some more so, some less so, but all of them have the same thing in common: they are responsible for themselves. Just as you are responsible for taking care of yourself and managing yourself, your pain management, and your coping strategies, so are they for themselves. It is not your job to fix the difficulties others have in dealing with the effects of your pain. It is not your job to cope for them or manage their emotional responses.

Of course, with those we are close to and who are likely to struggle the most with the effects of our chronic pain—partly through concern and love for us and partly through the big impact it has on their lives—it's natural to want to help them, to make it easier for them. Feeling responsible for another's inability to cope with our pain is very normal. It is my pain, after all. This person, my spouse or parent or child, is only affected by this, is only struggling with how to process their emotional response, because they are living with me, they care about me. It is an emotional reaction to me, so I should help them.

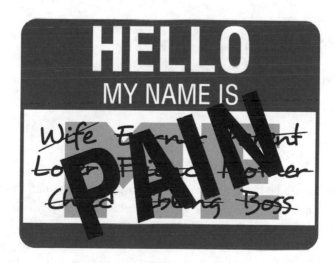

But you hear that? *Should. It's a reaction to me.* It's not and you shouldn't. It's a reaction to your pain, and you can help them, if you choose to. In many ways you might be best placed to help them, but certainly not at the cost of your own pain management. It is just as much their job to figure out how to cope with your pain as it is yours. Let me say that again: it is their job to manage their own emotional responses. You cannot take responsibility for that; you can try, as a good or caring person, to make it easier for them, to be empathetic and kind, but you can't take ownership. Aside from the fact you're not Superman, you're also not them. You're dealing with enough, and it's their responsibility. There is a fine line between helping someone through their process and trying to fix everything for them, and you have to walk that fine line.

Maintaining emotional and physical boundaries within relationships while experiencing chronic pain is extremely difficult, not just for you, but for your loved ones too. They will probably feel a reciprocal level of responsibility for taking care of you, helping you, managing your pain and health with you. Again, a certain level of give and take is always going to happen in any close relationship; supporting each other is what brings us closer together. That, however, is a very different notion from managing another person.

Relationships That Can Be Affected

Let's look at some of the relationships that can be affected by chronic pain:

Parents

Parents may find it the hardest to deal with a chronic pain ailment. Parents want their children to be safe and healthy, and chronic pain basically axes that. They may feel as if they've failed as a parent; they may expect themselves to be able to fix it for you, to make it better; they may be disappointed at your limitations and upset for you and themselves for their missed expectations. Depending on how old you are when experiencing chronic pain, their reactions may even make it worse. Many parents panic and feel helpless when their children are ill. Frustration, anger, depression, and catastrophizing are all common. This is very tough to deal with because our primary reaction is often to reassure. "Everything is fine." Even if it's not, you want to soften their reaction and help them cope.

Ultimately, the healthiest option is open, frank conversations about how you actually feel about your pain and the impact it is having on your life and accepting their emotional state for what it is. You should not have to hide your physical state to avoid their emotional reaction. They need to learn to deal with it. It is also really helpful to identify and discuss practical ways they can help and support you, so they don't feel so helpless, and so they know they are doing everything they can.

Children

Children can be insightful and susceptible to your emotional state. Expecting young children to live with the consequences of your chronic pain without help from you is clearly unfair and impractical. Especially with little ones, it can be very, very tough to explain what's happening and why, and to help children work through their reactions. But children are honest, up-front, and will usually take what you say at face value. Being matter-of-fact and owning your responses will help them with theirs. They need to know what they can do, if anything, to help you, and you need to know what helps them to feel safe and secure despite having a parent with chronic pain. Regulating your own emotional responses to your pain is never more important than when around children.

It is also important to note that parents experiencing chronic pain themselves are significantly more likely to catastrophize pain in their children. The fear that we have passed something along, that our kids will have to live with pain as we do—fear of ill-health in any of our loved ones—can be overwhelming. Maintaining perspective is very important, and ensuring your kids know the different types of pain and teaching them appropriate reactions will give them the best possible footing to deal with your and their own health.

Spouse

Spouses may have it the hardest. Did I already say that about parents? Well, it's true here too. Your spouse is the person who knows you best, who you live with, who is probably your primary caregiver, possibly who financially supports you, is the most familiar with your meds and doctors and routines and coping strategies, and has the greatest burden on them for managing. They are also the person you are closest with, have the weakest emotional and physical boundaries with, are intimate with, and, for most of us, expect to be treated as an equal partner by. See that? The trick there? They take care of you, support you, sometimes even physically support you, but you're still an equal. Yeah, right. Anyone who has lived with their partner through chronic pain knows that it rarely feels this way. Yeah, we're equal, aside from the fact that you do everything for me and do the majority of the work and earn all the money and take responsibility for helping me to manage my pain and and and. This is a very dangerous trap and possibly has the biggest impact on your sense of self, bigger than all of the other can'ts in your life. We want to support our partners, to love them, to take care of them, to help them cope, and they want to do the same, and fundamentally one of you is more physically capable than the other. So it's not a fair balance.

Fair and equal are not the same. Equal implies an even division of responsibility, 50/50. That may sound right, and even be right if both partners are absolutely the same, perfectly balanced in every way, but when they're not, it's a quick tip of the scale to unequal. Fair is a better way of looking at it; it may not be 50/50, but is it fair? Is it reasonable, given each person's abilities, to divide responsibility up that way? Fair might be 60/40. It might be 80/20 on a bad day. It can vary. Your partner may be ill some days and, on those days, you pick up the slack. It doesn't have to be a constant ratio, but a rationally, calmly considered evaluation of where each of you is and what is possible that day. Some days it might be equal, others not, but what is important is that both you and your spouse agree it is fair. Equal without due regard for circumstance makes no sense; fair can adapt to any circumstance.

Of course, the above assumes you have a partner whose reaction to your chronic pain is one of concern and over-helping. Many react very differently, with anger or disappointment or disbelief or depression. Their loss of expectation, their inability to regulate the mood changes that occur when you are in pain, their sense of helplessness can cause them to lash out, retreat, deny, give up, or blame themselves. Trying to help them through this is key, supporting them and letting them know they have a right to be angry, to be upset, to feel bad is important. But they don't have a right to be angry *with you*. They don't have a right to make you feel bad. They don't have a right to ignore your pain. And if they cannot cope with their emotional response to your pain, they need to know the effect that has on you. Both of your emotional boundaries are being violated in this situation and both of you need to take responsibility for protecting and managing your own selves before trying to help the other.

Both ends of the spectrum of reactions—overwhelming, desperate attempts to fix everything for you, and distance, blame, and ignoring the problem—are two opposite extremes, but both are caused by the same underlying issue: disappointment. One comes from disappointment for themselves and their expectations, and the other from disappointment for you. The balance, the healthy option, is in the middle: concern, empathy, and support, but also healthy detachment. There is a fine line between supporting you in your pain and trying to manage it for you, and this is the fine line your loved ones will have to walk.

Siblings

Siblings' responses to chronic pain can vary quite widely, depending on your relationship and at what age the chronic pain first started. When younger, siblings often take responsibility on themselves for helping you manage, but when they're older and independence has already been established, their help can be more limited. Many siblings feel a strong sense of loss when their partner-in-crime becomes limited in any way, and may feel bewilderment and a strong sense of survivor guilt. "Why not me?" They may also be confused and, occasionally, feel overshadowed if their brother/sister is suddenly getting all of the attention. This is not just a problem for the young—even adult siblings can feel threatened when ignored. It's important to make sure your sibling knows what's going on, is included in family discussions with your parents, and is given practical advice on how best to support you. The relationship you had before chronic pain is not gone; you are still siblings, and you can face the challenge of pain together.

Friends/Colleagues

Friends can have varying attitudes to your chronic pain depending on how long they've known you, the extent to which they are familiar with your health problems, and how much you rely on them. Acquaintances and distant colleagues are not really relevant, but close friends and those at work whom you rely on for support when you are in pain need to know what's going on. Asking for help from friends can bring you closer and is a perfectly reasonable choice, but it is fair that they know what's going on and how best to help you.

Sometimes your pain may affect your ability to participate with friends, to engage in plans with them; you may need to cancel at the last minute, change plans, or otherwise disappoint them. Some will react negatively to this, so it is important to be clear about what's happening. "I can't come because I'm having a bad pain day" is enough for most reasonable people to understand. They may be disappointed, but they will be disappointed that they can't see you, not disappointed in you. They know you have done nothing wrong. Apologizing for not being able to be with them is fair; apologizing for being in pain is not. And anyone who wants you to push through your pain for their convenience is not a friend. That sounds glib, but it's true. Cutting negative or selfish people out of your life is hard, but it will improve your ability to take care of yourself and help you to feel better.

Colleagues are trickier because they have fewer emotional ties with you and expect more consistency. Their disappointment or unwillingness to pick up your slack, to be understanding, or to care, will vary greatly, and you do not have a lot of choice about who these people are. All you can do is aim for fair; what is reasonable, what isn't, and if a colleague is unable to meet you at reasonable, speak to someone else, ask for another's help, or speak to a boss. You are not responsible for their inability to cope or desire not to have to deal with your pain. You are also not responsible for convincing them that your pain is real.

Trying to constantly explain yourself can lead to feeling overwhelmed that no one understands and reinforces the belief that there's something wrong with you. There isn't. I cannot say this enough: it is not your job to make everyone else understand. Explaining yourself over and over again to the same people is a choice, a cross you are choosing to bear. Learning how to say "I'm sorry you don't understand" and walking away is incredibly freeing, but it takes work to get there. It requires learning to care less about what others think of you than about taking care of yourself. Trust me, those people that are ignoring your boundaries or invalidating your experience are already way ahead of you in this, so don't feel guilty. They've put themselves first; you can too.

Caregivers

Caregivers have a hard time of it and in no way is the above intended to be a "fuck you, deal with it yourself" to any of them. But the best way to help them is to take care of yourself first and foremost. The better you are, the easier their lives will be.

Caregiving itself is a complex subject, and those living closely with you need to know what they're up against. Caregivers need to know the potential pitfalls and difficulties, and to develop their own coping strategies. Make it clear that their stress is their responsibility; make it clear that you will manage your pain if they will manage their stress associated with your pain. Dividing up labor in this way allows both to feel useful and capable without burdening the other unnecessarily. As mentioned above, you both have fine lines to walk between supporting one another and trying to take on the other's burden.

The addendum at the end of this book is intended for caregivers, to provide a brief overview of what they can expect and do. There are also a wide range of support groups, research reports, books, and articles intended to help caregivers living with someone in chronic pain. I highly recommend you and your loved ones prioritize learning from these; living normally with chronic pain is not just about you and you are not the only one who has to work at it. Those around you have to learn how to live normally as well.

Meeting New People

Meeting new people is an anxiety-inducing task; facing the thought of explaining yourself, quizzical looks, impertinent or even polite questions, all can raise a lump in your throat and the desperate desire to *avoid*. Learning to accept your body for what it is is the necessary first step toward making this less of a challenge and living life openly. You do not have to explain yourself, you do not have to justify yourself, and you are not responsible for other people's expectations. As they get to know you, they will learn your needs, but when starting out, you need to be able to state them openly and unapologetically.

Exercise:
Long-Term Mental Health Management

Sustained pain or illness will have an effect on mental health. There is no maybe about this. Mind and body are inextricably intertwined, and medicine is increasingly aware of this. Patients are treated as a whole and not as a collection of parts, and you too must consider yourself as a whole, with your emotional, psychological, and physical well-being all equally important.

Everything discussed in Part Two: Mind and Mood is part of the larger emotional and mental health consequences of long-term pain, but knowing about the issues and addressing them are two different things. Do not imagine that acknowledging and understanding is the same as managing. You can be fully aware of how your mental health has been affected by pain without being able to "fix" it all by yourself.

Pain psychologists, cognitive-behavioral therapists, psychologists, counsellors, and psychiatrists are extremely important resources that you cannot overlook. No matter what you need help with—whether it's using cognitive-behavioral training to reframe your emotional reactions to pain, or seeing a counsellor to talk through your loss of self-esteem, or visiting a psychologist to work through your feelings of anger and grief—there are resources available to you.

Many health insurance programs cover (at least partially) the cost of mental health care. When this isn't an option, there will be others. There are a lot of clinics that offer subsidized or free counselling; many of them have wait lists, but they are out there and putting your name down, even if you're not sure you need help, is great insurance against being caught out later.

So your exercise for Part Two: Mind and Mood is a simple one: get used to the idea of mental health care. Specifically, get used to the concept of *you* having to manage your mental health. Not as an emergency fail-safe when things get really bad, but as an ongoing part of your overall health care program. Just like going to the gym to keep your muscles healthy, taking care of your mental health should be an ongoing and proactive effort. And seeing a counsellor or seeking professional help for this care is just as normal and necessary as going to the doctor for any physical ailment you're not sure how to handle. Recognize this, and then internalize it, as it's vital for your long-term mental health management.

Part 3

TOOLS AND THERAPIES

Chapter 15

Medications

Medications can be a complex and baffling area, with many chronic pain sufferers using a combination of prescription and over-the-counter drugs to combat their symptoms and achieve day-to-day normality. There is also usually an element of trial and error in finding meds that work, and what works today may not work next month. Lastly, many pain meds are highly addictive, so dosing and proper use become very important. All of these factors—plus the fact that most of us are not chemists—can lead to a lot of misapprehension and confusion regarding what we can and should take.

One of the most under-utilized resources in health care is the pharmacist. For those many millions who visit only big-box pharmacies, seeing one of a number of interchangeable random people in white coats, giving your name and receiving a pill bottle with no explanation, then this is very understandable. Why would you engage with this stranger who acts as little more than a cashier in discussions about your health? Sadly, the rise of these enormous multi-function pharmacy retailers has made knowing your pharmacist seem like an old-fashioned notion, but it doesn't have to be. There are plenty of independent and smaller pharmacies still around. Even if you don't have a choice and have to go to a larger retailer for your prescriptions, there will usually be one or two supervising pharmacists on duty, present at set times, who you can ask to speak to and develop a rapport with.

Pharmacists are experts in medication—that's their whole job. They have gone to extensive educational lengths to become so. They usually know more than doctors about dosing, best practice for taking your medicine, potential complications, and drug interactions. Even if a medication has been prescribed by your trusted doctor, I would still recommend speaking to your pharmacist about it. Make sure they know everything you are on, over-the-counter meds included, and the issue being treated. They can advise on:

- Best practice taking medication (e.g. times of day, with/without food, in sequence or separate from other meds)

- Possible side effects

- Possible addictive qualities

- Possible interactions with other meds you may or may not be taking

- What to do if you miss a dose

- Expected efficacy, including a time window—especially if a slow-release pill

- Ramp-up time required (some drugs take several weeks to build up in your system before becoming fully effective)

All this information is needed for you to understand what you are taking, how to take it, and how to judge the efficacy of your meds. If it takes three weeks before your new prescription reaches effective levels in your system, there is no point in giving up on it after two weeks because it hasn't done anything yet. Doctors usually do not have the information or the time to share all of this detail with you, so speaking with your pharmacist should be considered a necessary second step, after initial prescription, before starting any new medication. They are also valuable resources on over-the-counter options, how to alleviate side effects, and combining multiple medications at once.

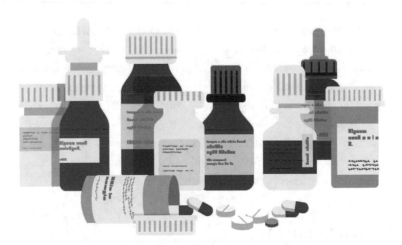

There will always be someone for you to talk to at whatever pharmacy you go to, because it's the law. A registered, fully trained pharmacist is required at all drug stores. You may need to ask to speak to them—you may need to come back if they are on break—but the awkwardness of asking a stranger about your prescriptions passes. Soon they will know you, will recognize you, and will be able to have an open and productive conversation with you (without prompting) to ensure you know everything you need to. For this reason, I highly recommend visiting only one location for your meds, and not buying them online. You risk missing out on one of the most beneficial health care relationships you can have as a chronic pain sufferer, one that doesn't even cost you anything extra.

Over-the-Counter Medications

There are a lot of over-the-counter pain medications and many people, with either temporary or chronic pain, utilize these before resorting to prescription meds or speaking with their doctor. It is important to be aware of the risks of continual use of these drugs, however, and to know what each can be best used for.

Ibuprofen

Ibuprofen is a non-steroidal anti-inflammatory drug (NSAID) for treating pain, fever, and inflammation. Commonly it is recommended for menstrual cramps, arthritis, and headaches and goes by several brand names, including Nurofen, Advil, Motrin, and Brufen. Store-bought ibuprofen comes in low doses (typically 200 mg, or 400 mg for extra strength) and dosing recommends taking no more than 1200 mg per day (for adults). Overuse of ibuprofen can increase the risk of heart, kidney, or liver failure, can worsen asthma, and can also cause stomach ulcers. To ameliorate the latter risk, take them with food and avoid alcohol.

Acetaminophen

Acetaminophen, also called Paracetamol or Tylenol, is used for pain and fever and is a common ingredient in many cold and flu medications. When combined with opioids in prescription meds, it can be a useful treatment for severe pain, but the over-the-counter versions are used for mild pain. Typical doses are 200–400 mg, with a maximum daily dose of 4,000 mg (orally, for adults). Side effects are minimal, but overdosing can cause liver damage.

Naproxen

Also known as Aleve, this strong NSAID painkiller relieves pain, swelling, and stiffness. It is very commonly used for back pain and arthritis but, like some of its NSAID counterparts, increases risk of stomach ulcers and as such should be taken sparingly and with food. It also interacts with alcohol. Side effects can include dizziness and headaches, and it can interact with other medications such as antidepressants, blood thinners, and heart medications. Maximum daily dose is 1,000 mg, usually in two tablets of 500 mg spaced apart.

Aspirin

Aspirin is the oldest drug in the NSAID family and has long been used for everything from pain to rheumatic fever. It is also commonly recommended to help prevent heart attacks. Like its NSAID brethren, continual use can increase the risk of stomach problems, and upset stomachs are the most common side effect of aspirin use. It is useful in the treatment of mild to moderate pain but is considered less effective than ibuprofen. Variants with additional ingredients are available to allow for quick release, but do not take more than three grams per day.

Topical Treatments

Many of the above active ingredients, and plenty of others, can be found in topical pain relief or anti-inflammatory treatments, such as Voltaren, Bengay, Icy Hot, Myoflex, Kalaya, and Aspercreme. These treatments can be applied directly to the painful area and as such are more targeted and less likely to cause internal side effects. Careful use is important, though— always follow the dosing and application instructions on the packet, wash your hands thoroughly after use, and stop using the product if you notice any skin irritation. Generally speaking, these topical treatments are not recommended for continual or long-term use, but rather to alleviate short-term or severe pain.

Prescription Painkillers

Most over-the-counter pain medications will contain a warning on the packet that says something like "do not use for more than a week in a row" or "contact your doctor if you use this product long-term." Chronic pain sufferers are generally advised not to rely (on a daily basis) on over-the-counter medications, as they have not been formulated for long-term continual use. Prescription medications are available for either safe daily use or to treat occasional, severe pain that needs something stronger than store-bought drugs.

There is an enormous variety in prescription pain medications and no way to cover them all in detail here, but the main categories are:

- Opioids

- NSAIDs (prescription strength)

- Antidepressants

- Corticosteroids

- Anti-seizure medications

- Muscle relaxants

Some of the above may not look like painkillers, but certain medications can have an effect on the way nerve signals are received by the brain and therefore, in low doses, reduce pain. Any of the above types should only be taken upon consultation with your doctor, taking into consideration every other medication you're on, and following dosing and usage guidelines carefully. There are multiple options within each category, so it may take a little while of trial and error with your doctor to find the best solution for you. Side effects or complications from your pain medication is a worry you can do without, so be prudent and only use what's recommended, regardless of how much pain you're in. It's also important to never, ever take another person's medications. You have no idea how they're going to interact with yours or your system, if they're in date, or even if they're safe.

A Note on Legality

We would be remiss if, when talking about chronic pain mitigation medications, we did not discuss the difficult and complicating factor of legality and availability. There are some common pain medications are that only legal or available in certain areas. An excellent example of this is medical marijuana—a substance over 3.5 million people in the US use but that is only partially legal. Many other countries across the globe have widely varying attitudes to marijuana, with some having an all-out ban and others allowing recreational use. Some people may have a doctor's prescription for it, others may quietly use it illegally but safely, others may not use it at all. A similar discussion can be had for certain opioids whose prevalence varies widely by geography.

It is unbelievably frustrating to have a working medication and not be able to travel with it. It is unbelievably frustrating to know of a potentially life-changing medication and not be able to try it because of the state you live in. It is unbelievably frustrating to be persecuted or targeted or in any way feel like a criminal for safely and privately using a medication that betters your life. This is yet another area where there is a frustrating lack of consistency and where you live (not to mention your skin color and wealth) can disproportionately affect your ability to access, use, and rely on potentially effective pain relief.

There is almost nothing positive to be said about this issue; it is very important for everybody to know their options. Have frank discussions with your doctors about what is and isn't available. Do not be afraid to ask about "taboo" substances—you are just asking! Wanting information is not a crime. Know your local laws, and know if they are changing soon. Know what to expect when using any substance, legally or otherwise, and always prioritize your safety. Be candid with family and close friends; the wide range of opinions of others may affect where and with whom you

can be appropriately medicated. Being up-front and honest can avoid
a lot of awkwardness and misunderstanding, as well as give you a good
indication of where and with whom you are comfortable and what risks
you are taking if traveling somewhere that will restrict your access to
your meds.

Medical marijuana can be and is enormously valuable for a lot of people,
but whether to try it, use it, or rely on it has to depend on your personal
priorities and the risks inherent to your situation, wherever you are.

Addiction and Perceived Drug-Seeking Behavior

A sad truth for many who have experienced long-term pain is that, at
some time or another, they have been accused of drug-seeking, of faking
their pain to gain access to narcotics. This feels awful, and it is absolutely
a complicated issue. For one thing, addiction *is* common among those
who have been using painkillers long-term. There is no blame or shame
on patients for this, and it by no means decreases the severity or existence
of their pain. Reliance on medication is a natural consequence of being
constantly in pain, and many drugs become less effective over time,
requiring ever-higher doses.

Add to this the fact that doctors can over-prescribe, leading to enormous
problems like the opioid crisis currently affecting the US. And, on top
of this, others can falsely present themselves as being in long-term pain
to obtain pills. With all of the stereotyping, hype, danger, judgment,
and nonsense that come with a system trying to help those in need and
simultaneously deny drugs to addicts, it's no surprise that those of us who
take medications long-term are in the crosshairs.

We're not going to talk about addiction in depth here. It's a huge topic,
and frankly one that's beyond my expertise. Professionals are available to
help those in long-term pain who are battling dosing and addiction issues,
and this is not something to fear bringing up with your doctor. Showing
willingness to talk about the potential dangers of long-term painkiller use

demonstrates to your physician how seriously you are taking your overall health, and it allows for open dialogue about all your options. This may involve counselling, addiction help, medication changes, or simply careful monitoring of your medication habits.

Openly discussing this topic with your doctor, however, is made a lot harder when so many of us have been falsely accused of faking our pain for drugs. Nothing is as upsetting as going to your doctor in good faith and being so harshly judged and ignored. Not only do you not receive the help you need, you're insulted and belittled into the bargain. There is no excuse for doctors who behave in this way—frankly, even if it were drug-seeking behavior, it should be met with compassion and kindness. As we discussed in Chapter 2, there's no point in seeing a medical professional who doesn't listen to you or care about you. How can you trust them with your health if they've just called you a liar to your face?

I wish I had always had the courage to stand up to this type of bully in the face of such brutal behavior, but it's not something most of us know how to do by instinct. Being accused of making it all up plays cruelly on the anxieties and fears inherent to pain and makes refuting such charges extremely difficult. It is especially tough as we do actually need something from the doctor—proper medical care. This is something we sorely want, and so we struggle to stay polite and reasonable even in the face of cruelty, in the hope they'll believe us and do their job.

As we've discussed at length, you can't make someone believe or understand you. There is no magic method for reacting when someone accuses you of drug-seeking behavior. You might get angry, you might get upset, you might want to leave. All of these are valid responses to such an attack. You might be able to get them to listen, you might not. All you can do is present the facts and go from there. But know this: your pain does not affect your right to being treated with dignity and kindness. Whatever the circumstances, whatever the situation, you as a person deserve to be given the same time and respect as everyone else. Do not accept less—doing so will reinforce your doctor's (and your own) belief that you are worth less.

Are You Kidding?

Sigh. Sounds really simple, right? Like so many of the topics covered in this book, it's a complex situation with easy-to-say, hard-to-do answers. Sure, I'll just be resolute in the face of discrimination. Sure, I'll never lose my shit in front of an asshole doctor or roommate or family member. Sure, I'll calmly set my boundary and put my needs first and always make the right choice and never backpedal or make a mistake, and everything will be alright. Well, no, you won't, because no one can, not all the time. No one is perfect, and it doesn't matter how well you know the theory or how well you understand the need to say or do the hard thing: sometimes you won't be able to. And that's okay. It isn't easy, and please don't take the black-and-white tone of the conversations here as a commentary on their easiness. They are *not easy*, they will take a lot of practice, of building up to your end goal in tiny steps, of work in progress, of mistakes and backward steps and frustration. This is natural—this is a normal part of growth. You can't hit the bullseye every time; what matters is that you're aiming for the right target.

And even when you do it right, it might not work out very well. It might even be temporarily worse, because you can't predict how someone else is going to react. This is disillusioning and difficult and makes you feel "What's the point?" What's the point in all my effort if it's making things worse? The point in the short term may be simply the act of putting yourself first, even if the results of doing so aren't perfect. You need to learn that your body and time and energy and self matter, regardless of your pain. And with time the act of putting yourself first becomes easier, and the results will come too. Life will improve. There is nothing so freeing as the perspective that comes with letting go of something that you were holding onto so tightly, only to realize it didn't matter anyway.

Exercise:
Connect with
Your Pharmacist

This exercise is a simple one. Write down your local pharmacy. Maybe this is the place you always go, maybe it's just the nearest to you. Maybe it's a new one down the street. Wherever it is, pick a single location you think you can reliably expect, from now on, to get your meds from. Write down its hours and make sure you will be able to drop off and collect prescriptions during those times. Google may be able to tell you the name of the pharmacist there—if so, great, write it down. If not, don't worry.

Go in and, at the pharmacy desk, ask to speak to the pharmacist. You may be told they're not in. You may be asked what it's regarding. Say you wish to discuss your medications with them, and leave your name and number if necessary. Explain that you have preexisting condition(s) and want to make sure you're taking everything safely and appropriately. The pharmacist may be in, in which case introduce yourself, state you are using their facility to fill your medication needs, and ask for a quick chat about what you're on. If they're not in, ask for a call back; if it's a place you've used before, they will have your details on file, but, if not, leave your name and number and prescription details, make sure you get the name of the pharmacist who will be contacting you, and have the discussion over the phone. The advantage of developing a relationship of this kind is that, quite quickly, you will be able to call the pharmacy with any questions and they will be able to help you over the phone, as they will know you and have your details in their system. A little work up-front can ensure a simple route to quick answers down the line.

All of this is designed to ensure you take what you need safely, but also to normalize a key aspect of your health care. Talking to your pharmacist should be and is a normal thing to do. They deal with medications all day every day; there is no shame in using their expertise. Removing the awkwardness, the embarrassment, the self-consciousness of such a vital component of pain management is a big step toward making it everyday and routine. It's not mystical, it's just chemistry, and the quicker you learn how to speak about it and treat it as such, the easier it will be to understand, manage, and control your medications.

Chapter 16

Mindfulness and Meditation

O f all the concepts tackled in this book, I have found this one the hardest to write about. You hear people say "Breathe through the pain" all the time—on TV, at the hospital, at yoga. Instructions to breathe have become so ubiquitous and meaningless that writing about it here seemed pointless. Most of my life, when I have heard the recommendation to breathe, I have felt a deep spiritual need to cause physical harm to the moron saying it. Like a pregnant woman who can scream and be violent during childbirth when told to calm down, I want to lash out at the uselessness of the suggestion. But. Argh, but. It's not all bullshit. It's the go-to suggestion because it does actually help. I sort of wish it didn't, it seems like such a nonsense form of self-control, and would almost wish it away for the intellectual satisfaction of being right, if only it wouldn't mean losing a primary coping strategy.

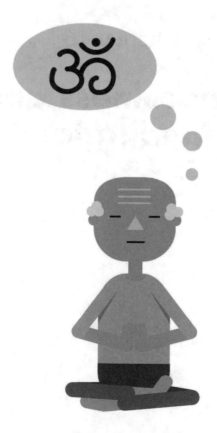

Breathing and meditation go hand in hand. Meditation doesn't have to be anything about spirituality, religion, energy flows, vibrations, ley lines, karma, chakras, the cosmos, or any of the other vague nonsense you've probably heard if you've ever done a yoga class. Meditation can be, and in its purest form is, about self-awareness and achieving a calm, clear-minded state without suffering.

Pain Versus Suffering

There is an old Buddhist quote: "Pain is inevitable, suffering is not." Pain of any kind is unavoidable in life, but a significant aspect of the effect it has on us comes not from the pain itself, but from our interpretation of the pain, the way we deal with it. Pain is an experience; suffering is the reaction to that experience—an emotional reaction we can control versus the physical reality of the pain we cannot. Typically, definitions state that pain has a purpose, while suffering does not. Chronic pain does not necessarily have a purpose, so the simplistic definition does not hold up here, but the truth of suffering's uselessness remains. Suffering achieves nothing. It does nothing. We already know something is wrong because of the pain. Suffering is a futile, pointless addition that only heightens pain, makes us feel worse emotionally, and lengthens the whole ordeal.

You can control how much you suffer. Suffering is a choice, and with practice you will be able to control whether it affects you or not. A big part of suffering comes from the emotional attachment to pain. We want to fight it, we want to cry, it disappoints us, it causes guilt and feelings of inadequacy. But does it really? Is it the pain doing that, or your brain responding to the pain? The pain is just pain—ow, my leg hurts. There are neurons firing electrical signals from my leg up my spine to my brain. That's it. Everything else is your addition. You are not your leg and your leg does not define you. Once you can detach yourself and your emotional experience from the pain, then you can see it for what it is: it's just pain. It doesn't mean anything bigger, it doesn't have a mind of its own (although it may seem like it), it doesn't have a personality or motive or opinions or anything else. It's just pain. It's just a sensation, one of many. It can be a *just*.

Mindfulness

Being a smart observer of your own body, knowing the types of pain, being able to recognize your responses—basically everything we have talked about so far—is part of a bigger picture to reduce suffering through mindfulness. We can't fix the pain, but we can change how we are with it, giving ourselves more room to live our lives. Mindfulness is simply the awareness of ourselves, an ancient and really simple form of meditation. Notice what's going on in your body, but don't let it own you. Recognize it, understand it, accept it, but don't become it. Don't let it be you. It's not you, it's just a pain in your leg. There is so much else going on that it does not deserve all of your attention or behavior.

Mindfulness as a form of treatment for chronic pain is now considered so effective that some hospitals are actually prescribing mindfulness programs to patients. Clinical trials show that it reduces chronic pain by 57 percent. Brain imaging shows it soothes brain patterns associated with pain and, over time and with practice, can permanently change the brain's response to pain, decreasing pain frequency and intensity. If you heard of a medication, a pill, that cost nothing, was risk-free, and was as effective as this, I'm pretty sure you'd take it.

Mindfulness, the practice of it, is no more complicated than breathing and being aware of your body. We discuss retraining the nervous system in depth later, but mindfulness is really much the same thing. Learn how to breathe deeply (actual deep belly breaths, not gasps of air) and calmly observe how your body feels all over. Examine every part of you and think: how does this feel? What's really going on? Ignore outside distractions and just listen to your body. Doing so allows you to insert space between your pain and your reaction to your pain, thereby circumventing the negative cycle of pain-negative emotional reaction-tension-pain. Your pain becomes a single, quantifiable mass, instead of a great sprawling emotional monster that touches and infects everything, and, with that, your ability to move past it increases and your pain decreases. Your brain learns that pain is not the be-all and end-all of your body and, by teaching your brain this, it no longer goes into hyperdrive with every pain but is able to say "Yeah, okay, this hurts, but there's a lot else going on as well" and effectively turn the dial of your pain down. What starts as conscious practice becomes, over time, an automatic response. No, this is not the magic cure I promised none of you would get at the start of the book, but it can be very, very helpful in calming your nervous system down. It's not a solution, just a valuable tool. Removing suffering significantly ameliorates even the worst pain. It also gives you the room to figure out what you need to do when you're overwhelmed. Don't know where to start, struggling to cope? Calming yourself and resetting, going back to basics, is a part of mindfulness, and often the fastest way to get yourself back on track.

In the bibliography at the end of this book I have included a few resources for more information on the practice of mindfulness techniques. Needless to say, there are many, but the ones I share are based on scientific studies and reviewed by peers. There are also apps, videos, and websites dedicated to this field, as well as practitioners and teachers all over who can provide in-person assistance if this is a route you wish to explore.

A Note on Religion

I've deliberately avoided talking about religion here, because the way religious belief and pain interact is such a deeply personal issue, and may depend greatly on the religion in question, past experiences, personal religious practices, cultural expectations that come with a shared religion, and so on. What I will say is this: meditation and mindfulness are not in conflict with religious practices. In fact, for many, prayer is a form of meditation. It involves the same steps: considering one's situation, acknowledging flaws and mistakes, and surrendering oneself. Prayer, just like meditation, can be extremely comforting and relaxing and can give you room to accept yourself and your situation. Do not let stereotypes or assumptions about meditation and how it speaks to your own religion cloud your judgment; you can have both—they have the same root, and they complement each other well.

Exercise:
Simple Meditation Practices

Task 1: Box Breathing

Practicing deep breathing is easy but important. Conscious effort is required when beginning, so that your body can learn the routine and its effects, the better to react and follow that routine in times of stress. You do not want the first time you attempt deep breathing to be when you're in severe pain. Practice, get good at it, and your body will know what to do when it needs it.

Imagine a square. Each side of the square is measured in time, three seconds per side. Breathe in along one side of the square, for three seconds. Hold your breath along the next side of the square, for three seconds. Breathe out along the next side, three seconds. Then hold again along the last side, back to your starting point, for three seconds. The aim is to pace each breath and hold equally, a long three seconds, with the breath in and out being consistent. Fill your lungs in those three seconds and empty them again in the following three. Repeat for five minutes. Just close your eyes and envision the box and breathe along its sides, over and over again, letting your mind focus on nothing but the box and the air expanding and contracting your body. Let the air breathe you; feel your chest and belly expand and collapse with each breath.

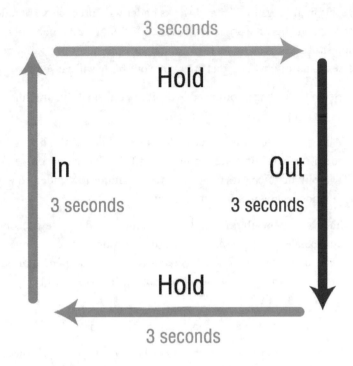

Task 2: Progressive Muscle Relaxation[5]

You can consciously and deliberately relax all the muscles in your body to release tension and ease pain. This is a well-known and often-used technique. Read the basic instructions below for a guideline, but I recommend listening to an audio clip of the instructions during your first few practices for simplicity. There are a ton of free audio clips and videos online that follow this same basic technique, and the name given above is the official one.

---

5   Harold Cohen, "Progressive Muscle Relaxation," Psych Central, last modified October 8, 2018, https://psychcentral.com/lib/progressive-muscle-relaxation.

Again, this method gets easier and works better with practice, so practice. Over time it will become possible to use this technique even in highly stressful situations, such as during hospital visits, to minimize pain and decrease the harmful effects that stress on your body will cause.

1. Begin by finding a comfortable position, either sitting or lying down, somewhere quiet.

2. Allow your attention to focus only on your body. If you begin to notice your mind wandering, gently bring it back to yourself without judgment. It's totally normal for minds to wander, so when you notice it happening, just refocus on your body.

3. Take a deep breath through your abdomen, hold for a few seconds, and exhale slowly. As you breathe, notice your stomach rising and your lungs filling with air. Take your time and just spend a minute or two breathing and noticing your breathing. Feel your body already relaxing.

4. As you go through each step, keep breathing normally.

5. Tighten the muscles in your forehead by raising your eyebrows as high as you can. Hold for about five seconds and abruptly release, feeling that tension fall away. Pause, feeling the relaxation seep through your forehead, and breathe.

6. Now smile widely, feeling your mouth and cheeks tense. Hold for about five seconds, and release. Pause. Let the relaxation spread across your cheeks; feel your jaw gently open. Concentrate only on the feeling of your lower face softening. Breathe. Pause for five to ten seconds.

7. Next, tighten your eye muscles by squinting your eyelids tightly shut. Hold for about five seconds, and release. Pause for five to ten seconds, concentrating only on the weight of your eyes in their sockets.

8. Gently pull your head back as if to look at the ceiling. Hold for about five seconds, and release, feeling the tension melting away. Pause, breathing calmly. Feel the weight of your relaxed head and neck sink back.

9. Keep breathing deeply, evenly.

10. Now, tightly, but without straining, clench your right fist and hold this position for about five seconds. Pause. Feel the tension in your right forearm and hand. Feel that buildup of tension. You may even visualize that set of muscles tightening. Release and enjoy the feeling of limpness spreading across your right hand and up your arm.

11. Breathe in…and breathe out…

12. Tense your entire right arm. Feel the taut muscles, strain against them. Hold for about five seconds, and release. Pause and breathe. Let your arm be heavy, feel it sink.

13. Repeat the process, first with your left hand, and then with your whole left arm.

14. Now lift your shoulders up as if they could touch your ears. Hold for about five seconds, and quickly release, feeling their heaviness. Pause, releasing all of the tension, lowering your shoulders as far as they will go. Keep breathing.

15. Tense your upper back by pulling your shoulders back, trying to make your shoulder blades touch. Hold for about five seconds, and release. Relax your back, let it melt into the bed or chair supporting you. Visualize it melting. Pause in the relaxation.

16. Tighten your chest by taking a deep breath in; hold for about five seconds, and exhale, blowing out all the tension. Breathe deeply, allowing your chest to relax naturally.

17. Now tighten the muscles in your stomach by sucking in and clenching your abdominals. Hold for about five seconds, and release.

18. Feel the limpness across your upper body. Feel the heaviness and weight of it, the ground or chair or bed you are on supporting you like it is pushing upwards against you.

19. Tense your entire right leg and thigh. Contract the muscles tightly. Hold for about five seconds…and relax. Feel the tension melting away from your leg. Let it fall heavy, melt, and relax.

20. Flex your right foot, pulling your toes toward you and feeling the tension in your calf. Hold for about five seconds…and relax, feel the weight of your leg sinking down.

21. Curl your toes under like they are talons gripping a branch. Tense your whole foot. Hold for five seconds, then release.

22. Repeat with your left leg, left foot, and left toes.

23. Now imagine a wave of relaxation slowly spreading through your body, beginning at your head and going all the way down to your feet. Each wave feels warm and comforting. Your body is completely relaxed. Feel the weight of your relaxed body. Keep breathing deeply.

24. As you breathe, notice your stomach rising and your lungs filling with air. Take your time and just spend a minute or two breathing and noticing your breathing.

25. As you exhale, imagine the tension in your body being released and flowing out of your body.

26. Feel your body fully relaxed now. You are done and feeling completely relaxed.

Chapter 17

Alternative Therapies

Alternative therapies are a divisive topic. Even what is considered alternative can lead to blazing rows and awkward silences at dinner parties. Cultural and regional practices vary a lot, and what's considered health care and what faux medicine depends on where you live, who you're with, and what you're used to. It also changes over time. Keeping track of what you're supposed to seriously consider and what you're supposed to laugh at can be exhausting and, frankly, a waste of your time. The majority of therapies that fall in the gray area between strict medicine and placebos are subjective. The exact shade of gray depends partly on current societal views and partly on you.

I really don't care if a particular therapy works because of a placebo effect or because of a knowable, traceable medical effect. The result is the same. If I feel better, I feel better. If that is replicable through continued use of a particular therapy, then that's a win. End of story. At some point, the only reason to care why it works is if that can give you new information about how to better treat or understand your pain. If it can, great! If not, well, it's still a win—because you feel better. The only other factor scientific legitimacy should have on your decisions about which therapies to use relates to insurance coverage. Prevailing opinion on the validity of a particular therapy does have an impact on what is covered by health care providers and insurance carriers, and this may determine what you can afford to try. Unfortunately, there's not a lot you can do about this, other than consider switching insurance carriers to one who offers more coverage, if that is an option for you.

Generally, though, I advocate ignoring everyone else when it comes to "legitimacy" and doing whatever works for you. You are the only person in your body and feeling your pain. Some therapies may make you uncomfortable even if they are medically sound, and some may make you relax even if they have no scientific basis. So try a bunch, see what works for you. An enormous amount of pain management is about relaxing and retraining your nervous system, and a big portion of that is in your head. So if it comforts, relaxes, relieves, or otherwise benefits you, then it doesn't matter whether there is a defensible scientific reason why. Do not accept other people's judgments about what makes you more comfortable—do what works for you. You do not have to explain yourself.

The sentence "It helps in my pain management" should be enough to silence anyone but the most obnoxious know-it-all.

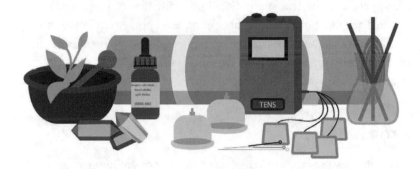

There are a lot of alternative therapies to try, some of which you may be familiar with, some of which may seem very alien. The list below is not exhaustive and is not a recommendation; it is simply a collection of some of the most commonly available alternative therapies today. And note that some of these you may not think of "alternative." You may look at the below list and find something that, where you are, is practiced by doctors and is considered on par with the strict definitions of modern medicine. As we discussed above, this is regional and variable, and what's practiced by MDs in one place is not necessarily considered a medical service in other countries, and may not be subject to the same regulations, stringency, or standards. So knowing your own local standards is wise.

Some of the below therapies may interest you, some you may know already work for you, some you may think are nonsense. But know that there are a lot of options out there, whatever your comfort level. Trying something new may open a door for you, or it may be a waste of your time. Only you can decide how to prioritize your time and money.

Acupuncture

Acupuncture relies on the use of thin needles to puncture the body, stimulate nerves, and relieve pain. It is an ancient form of therapy and still widely debated, with little empirical evidence but many adherents; it is said to be especially useful in the treatment of chronic pain conditions. It can cause some mild bruising and achiness, though, so be warned. This common form of treatment is offered through a lot of alternative therapy clinics, as well as at traditional physiotherapists. Properly certified acupuncturists need to have completed proper schooling and pass an examination before becoming registered, though there are a lot of unregistered practitioners too. Do your research and visit a clean, reputable clinic if attempting acupuncture.

Aromatherapy

Aromatherapy uses scents from plants and plant oils to improve physical and psychological well-being. It is often used to alleviate anxiety, depression, headaches, pain, and sleep troubles. Aromatherapists use oils through topical application, water immersion, inhalation, or massage, so prepare to get a little messy. Patients with sensitive skin or allergies should do their research before attempting aromatherapy, as certain oils are known to have potentially adverse effects.

Ayurveda

Ayurveda is a system of medicine and set of spiritual beliefs originating from the Indian subcontinent and based on the idea that all areas of life impact health. It is the world's oldest health care system and has many roots and specialties, but relies on treating the person as whole, assuming a person's health is based on three aspects of them: physical presence, mental existence, and personality. It uses a medieval classification of tissue types within the body, and problems are diagnosed through the five senses. Ayurveda is contraindicated for many and some of its medicaments have been shown to contain potentially dangerous levels of toxic heavy elements.

Bowen Techniques

The Bowen Technique is a non-invasive therapy whereby certain points in the body are targeted with gentle rolling movements to help the body balance, repair, and reset itself. The movements used are very distinctive and manipulate soft tissues in a specific way, over a very small area. In theory, Bowen therapy treats musculoskeletal and neurological problems; practitioners are not medical professionals.

Chiropractic

Chiropractors are relatives of the osteopath, focusing specifically on the diagnosis and treatment of mechanical disorders of the musculoskeletal system, in particular the spine. A chiropractor will use hands-on spinal manipulation to align the body's musculoskeletal structure and relieve pain. Many patients experience short-term relief but no long-term advantage. Chiropractors do not hold medical degrees but are usually specially educated and regulated. There are many chiropractors available, as this is a widely used form of treatment, so make sure if visiting one that they are registered with a professional body

Craniosacral Therapy

Craniosacral therapy is almost a form of massage, but it focuses specifically on manipulating and massaging the skull to help harmonize the central nervous system. It uses gentle touch, almost exclusively on the skull but occasionally on the spine also, to promote the flow of cerebrospinal fluid. In theory, this relieves tension and stress, and some claim it can cure other ailments (cancer is a notable example of a disproven claim). For those with amorphous chronic pain conditions, this may be a novel therapy addressing the nervous system specifically.

Crystal Healing

Crystals are considered, by some, to contain certain types of energy that, when held against or moved around the body, can promote physical and spiritual wellness. Different crystals have different properties in this regime and can be used to promote a variety of results. Crystal healing is absolutely not a scientific method or in any way medically sound, but for those believing in it, it can help improve mood.

Cupping

Cupping therapy involves a therapist placing special cups on your skin to create suction; it is intended to help with pain, inflammation, and circulation and acts as a form of massage. It is most often practiced on patients who are otherwise healthy—particularly athletes—and is not recommended for those with preexisting conditions due to the potential for complications.

Electromagnetic Therapy

Electromagnetic therapy has many names (bioelectricity, magnetobiology); it uses machinery to pulse electromagnetic fields through the body, with the aim of these energy waves changing the way your body responds to pain. Both electrical and magnetic energy exist naturally within the body already, and some forms of electromagnetic equipment are in common use in medicine—for example, defibrillators for restarting a stopped heart. TENS units are becoming more widely used to treat localized pain by attaching electrodes to a certain part of the body and pulsing small amounts of energy through it. Machines also exist to help with circulation, tissue damage, and more. There is a variety of evidence that suggests this form of therapy has potential to ease pain in the short term and redefine how the body copes with pain in the longer term.

Homeopathy

Homeopathy is an alternative medicine predicated on the notion that substances that cause illness in healthy people can be used to cure similar symptoms in sick people. It relies on the body's ability to heal itself when introduced to a foreign substance. Despite being a widely discredited form of medicine (often referred to as "herbal" medicine), many people continue to rely on it. The substances used are minuscule doses of naturally occurring plant, animal, and mineral extracts, heavily diluted with water. Almost anyone can be a homeopath, although several large organizations exist which accept members and provide education and professional development.

Hydrotherapy

Hydrotherapy uses water for the treatment of pain. Temperature and pressure of the water can be varied to stimulate blood circulation and encourage mobility. Hydrotherapy covers a range of techniques, including mineral baths, underwater massage, hot tubs, underwater jets, and cold plunges, either for the whole body or just a part. Its primary goal is as a medium for delivering heat and cold to facilitate thermoregulatory reactions in the body. It has long been used as a tool in burn and wound treatment in hospitals but can also be used as an all-purpose wellness tool or to stimulate physiological responses in a specific area of the body.

Hypnosis

Hypnosis is a state of consciousness that requires reduced peripheral awareness and inward-focused attention; it is associated with a heightened degree of suggestibility. A hypnotist will attempt to put you to sleep by relaxing your awareness and clearing your mind, thereby producing a susceptible state in which he or she can make suggestions for relaxation and comfort, some of which can be carried over into day-to-day life through the use of cues or triggers to recall a relaxed state. There is actually an increasing amount of evidence that suggests this may be a replicable form of treatment for chronic pain patients. There exist many quacks in this field, so do your research before putting yourself under someone else's control. Bear in mind that good hypnotherapists will teach patients how to train themselves, sometimes even providing tapes for use at home, to allow patients to self-hypnotize at will.

Kinesiology Taping

Kinesiology tape is a form of tape that, when applied properly, lifts skin and creates space between the muscle and dermis layers, thereby relieving pressure on swollen or injured muscles. It also allows muscles to move more freely and encourages blood flow. Many physiotherapists use kinesiology tape at the end of treatments to hold a muscle or joint in place, and it is freely available in stores, with instructions provided both with the tape and online on how to properly apply it across the body. It is in common use for those experiencing short-term or temporary muscular issues, but is not a long-term solution for pain.

Magnet Therapy

Magnet therapy uses magnets to provide weak magnetic fields around the body to promote healing. Magnetic bracelets are quite common nowadays and claim to cure all sorts of physical and psychological problems. A cousin of electromagnetic therapy, the magnets in magnet therapy are very weak, so although magnetism does already exist in the body and could in theory be affected by magnetic fields, the actual magnets used are too weak to create any measurable change in a body's function.

Massage Therapy

Massage therapy is actually quite a broad term, as there are many forms of massage, from Swedish to deep tissue to shiatsu to hot stone, and many more. Massage can technically be performed by anyone, but most reputable massage therapists have gone to school, passed certification, and are registered with a regulatory body. Massage involves the kneading and rubbing of muscles and joints to relieve tension and pain; patients will often be asked to partially undress for proper contact with the skin. Oils may sometimes be used. Massage can be relaxing and sometimes painful, so it's important to discuss your pain thresholds and any problem areas before beginning treatment.

Myofascial Release

Myofascial release is a growing area of study, almost a subset of massage, that treats musculoskeletal immobility and pain caused by contracted muscles through stretching the connective tissues across muscles (known as fascia) to release them. It also aims to improve circulation. This is a hands-on technique offered by physiotherapists, massage therapists, and, in some cases, specially trained physical therapists. It is not fully regulated, and efficacy can vary depending on the underlying cause of the tension and pain.

Naturopathy

Naturopathy is more a system of alternative medicine than a single technique. It relies on the idea that medical problems can be treated without the use of drugs or medical intervention through proper regulation of diet, exercise, and massage. It is a totally non-invasive philosophy that aims to promote the body's own ability to heal. The beliefs behind naturopathy have gone in and out of style and are currently seeing a resurgence in North America. Patients seeing a naturopath may expect to be given dietary advice, natural supplements, homeopathic medicine, physical treatments such as massage and acupuncture, and lifestyle counselling.

Nutritional Therapy

Nutritionists (also known as dietitians) are experts in food; usually requiring a degree and professional accreditation, a nutritionist can work with a patient to identify unhealthy eating habits and work collaboratively with you, within your health requirements, to see that you follow the healthiest diet possible to ensure maximum wellness. This might include setting diet plans, providing recipes, educating on nutrition, and helping you understand your weight.

Osteopathy

Osteopathy emphasizes the treatment of medical issues through massage and manipulation of bones, joints, and muscles, with the intent of removing tensions and restrictions in the vascular, neural, and biomechanical systems of the body. Its aim is to promote the body's own healing properties in a drug-free, non-invasive way. During a visit to the osteopath, a patient will be massaged and moved about to increase mobility. Expect to be asked to demonstrate stretches, and to be a little sore after appointments. Osteopaths can be doctors or surgeons, but they can also be non-medical manual therapists. The vast majority of alternative treatment facilities offering osteopathy do so using non-medical professionals. Interesting fact: osteopathy in this form is actually the fastest-growing health care profession in the US.

Physiotherapy

Physiotherapy comprises a broad range of treatment performed by professionals to treat musculoskeletal conditions such as sprains, muscle and joint pain, injuries, posture problems, arthritis, and reduced mobility. Physiotherapists must complete extensive schooling, accreditation, and regulation to practice and are often referred to by physicians for rehabilitation care. They use a combination of manual manipulation, massage, ultrasound, heating/cooling, electrotherapy, and exercise programs to treat and ease pain and injury. Most people assume that physiotherapists only treat one-off injuries, for example when recovering from a broken leg, but in fact physiotherapists often work on an ongoing basis with those experiencing long-term mobility issues to increase their range of motion and decrease pain.

Reflexology

Reflexologists massage the hands and feet, without oils, to produce an effect in other areas of the body. It relies on the premise that all areas of the body can be mapped from the hands and feet, and that pressing on certain areas of the hands or feet will create the desired effect in the associated area of the body. There is no medical evidence to support reflexology, and regulatory and educational requirements vary widely by country and state, but many devotees respond primarily to its overall relaxing effect.

Finding One That Works

The disadvantage of many chronic pain conditions is their vagueness; similarly, many alternative therapies can be considered pretty vague, treating a range of conditions and symptoms with varying efficacy. Almost any clinic providing some form of alternative therapy will tell you that their services could "potentially" help improve your condition, but, by their very nature, they cannot guarantee anything. It is important to know what to expect, to seek qualified and registered professionals in whichever disciplines you choose to try, and to be open and honest with them about your physical status.

Here are some simple guidelines:

- Be clear that you have specific goals and desires for your therapy and will be monitoring your progress.

- Some therapists state up-front that multiple sessions are required to notice progress, and this should be expected, but run from anyone promising miracle cures or asking you to pay for a set number of sessions up-front. (I cannot drive around my relatively small town without seeing multiple billboards asking "Chronic Pain? X therapy can make you pain-free!" As a point of principle, I never go near these clinics).

- Give it a fair shot, and give your therapist feedback (it should be remembered that, as each of us is unique, it may take your therapist a little while to get to know your body and how it reacts) so they know what is working and what isn't.

- Be prepared to move on. Some therapies may just not work; in some cases, it might be a particular therapist who isn't adapting to your needs very well. In either instance, know you can ask questions, expect clear answers, and ask for referrals or recommendations if you feel the particular person you are seeing is not a good fit but aren't ready to give up on the method just yet. The internet is a great resource for what's available locally and usually has some good tips on the best practitioners, with reviews and helpful advice.

- Expect reputable businesses to provide information on their data privacy rules (required by all companies collecting health information).

- Expect your initial session to include a lengthy medical questionnaire and a discussion about your existing conditions and past illnesses. This should occur any time something new is tried, and your therapist should be prepared to have open, frank dialogue with you about benefits and risks associated with each new therapy or technique.

- If you are interested in trying a treatment but some aspect of it makes you uncomfortable, say so. For example, many people have difficulty with the nudity aspect of massage therapy. Talking this over with the therapist before making an appointment is a great idea, as they have probably encountered it before and may be able to provide suggestions or modifications to allow you to still try it out.

Some people go for a manicure every week. Some people get their hair cut or colored regularly. Others go to the gym fanatically, or buy expensive clothes, or wear fancy perfume, or shave every day, or wear a lot of makeup, or count calories, or any number of normal and pretty routine things, some of which count as health care and some of which just make people feel better. Making one or more alternative therapies part of your life as a pain management tool is exactly the same; less common, maybe, but no less valid and no less normal. If it makes you feel better, makes you more comfortable in your body, and in any way improves your pain or mobility, that is the only metric that counts.

Exercise:
Rating Therapies

From the list of therapies above, make a list in the following format and slot each therapy in as you see fit:

Have Already Tried	Want to Try	Do Not Want to Try

For those in the first column, go through each one and rate the success of the treatment you received by noting, from one (no benefit) to ten (brilliant), both short-term improvement and long-term benefits (if any).

Example:

Have already tried: Massage

Short-term benefit: 8/10—significant improvement for several days after each session.

Long-term benefit: 1/10—results faded with time and required ongoing treatment for continued benefits.

Now rate the cost and time required for these therapies, from one (very costly) to ten (no cost at all):

Therapy: Massage

Time cost: 8/10—an hour a week but can adapt to my schedule as needed.

Financial cost: 2/10—expensive and not covered by insurance.

Add the numbers for each individual therapy together like so:

Short-term benefit + long-term benefit + time cost + financial cost

Then rank the therapies you have tried. Simplistically, those with a higher score got you more benefit for less cost, and those with a lower score got you less or no benefit for higher cost. You can also compare across categories—for example, a therapy might be costly in the short term but provide better long-term benefits. You can use these metrics to compare therapies and make rational decisions about where to concentrate your efforts.

Now, for those in the middle column, "Would Like to Try," list them in priority order. Research local providers (the internet and support groups are a great resource for this) and for each therapy write down:

Therapy name
Chosen provider 1
Chosen provider 2
Cost
Expectations for improvement

Try each therapy on your list in turn, one at a time (trying multiple new therapies at once may confuse results, as you won't be able to tell which benefit came from where). Give each one a set amount of time, e.g. a month of solid attempt, before evaluating the therapy using the grading system above. Add it to your list of already-trieds and see where it ranks. Is it worth continuing? Is it time to move on and try the next on the list?

Eventually, you'll run out of options from the first two columns. Then it is time to reevaluate whether your stance has changed on any from the third. You can also research other alternative therapies and add them to the list above. The aim here is to understand your range of options and have a clear idea of which among those you've tried is worth pursuing, for you. Investigating your insurance coverage can also help establish what is reasonable to have in your "to try" list, as those with little or no financial cost are probably easier long-term solutions.

Chapter 18

Retraining Your Nervous System

A lot of what we have talked about so far has, either directly or indirectly, served an important purpose: helping to retrain your nervous system. This is a pretty weird concept, but one that is helpful to become familiar with, not only unconsciously as you go about your daily life, but also as a conscious, concerted effort.

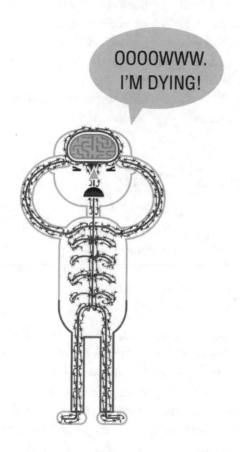

Being in chronic pain is like having your nervous system dialed up to a hundred, all the time. Even when you're not in physical pain, your body starts to anticipate it, to tense or flinch and become hyper-aware of how everything feels. It is easy, in this state, to want to avoid physical stimuli of any kind, regardless of how it *might* make us feel, simply because, by tensing in anticipation, our bodies put us on the path to pain. Physical stimuli are known to us as the precursors of pain, so why not avoid them?

Well, the nervous system is a strange beast. Being hyper-aware all the time is not healthy and will not help minimize or ease pain. Being hyper-sensitive to pain does not help. And avoiding physical stimuli can be a lot like avoiding life, which is also not healthy and will exacerbate the emotional consequences of pain. So what can we do? Our bodies are hypersensitive to pain and everything else, and the negative stimuli that have caused this are not really under our control. Okay, so most of us will try to ensure that we don't get punched, or fall down the stairs, or anything else obvious that will hurt, but the day-to-day pains of living in our body are usually pretty hard to control. There is something you can control, though, one really significant input to your nervous system: positive physical stimuli.

Positive Stimuli

Positive stimuli are, basically, actions or sensations that feel nice to you. They may be relaxing in the moment, they may be exciting, they may be calming, they may be surprising; touch is the typical basis for positive stimuli, for the obvious reason that it is through this sense that we perceive pain. There are a myriad of possibilities for something to feel good in your body, and everyone is different.

Oxytocin is a wonderful hormone (commonly called the "love hormone") released by the pituitary gland during times of pleasure (and, in some cases, pain) that has the effect of making you feel, well, lovely. Evolutionarily, it serves an important purpose during childbirth, but let's assume you want some without going into labor. It can be released in response to massage, physical touch, warmth, and low-intensity electrical stimulation, and when it is released it increases pain threshold, calms stress, regulates behavior, and increases function of the internal organs. It's basically a wonder drug, and it is safe and freely available within your own body. It will make you feel better. So how do you get some? Engaging in positive physical stimuli is how; some examples of positive stimuli are:

- Massage

- Caresses and gentle touch

- Stretching or releasing tension

- Sex

- Cuddles (human or animal)

- Warmth

- Water immersion

- Hot tubs

- Manicures and pedicures

- Head massage

- Haircut/style/wash

- A gentle breeze

- Food intake

- Sunshine

- Lotions or creams to soothe skin

- Music

- A bath or shower

- Swinging/rocking motion (e.g. on a hammock or swing)

Emotional Benefits

It may seem like enough to you to just avoid pain. Do the things that minimize pain and leave it at that. Why go to all the extra effort to feel positive physical stimuli as well? I'm busy just existing over here! But experiencing positive physical sensations in your body is vital. The reason this is so important, aside from the release of helpful hormones, is that it teaches your body and your brain a few really crucial things:

1. You have the capacity to feel physical pleasure.

2. Not every physical stimulus is bad or will hurt.

3. You have control over aspects of how you feel physically.

4. You have the ability to relax and quiet your nervous system.

Knowing that you can feel physically good in your body is not a concept to be underestimated. I'm going to repeat that, as it is so important. Look at point number one again: you have the capacity to feel physical pleasure. A lot of us in chronic pain go day to day trying to feel as not-crappy as possible. All of the focus and attention is on managing, and as such our bodies become, to some extent, the enemy. We have to deal with them, cope with them, manage them, suffer them. But there is more. You have the ability to feel good in your body—to actually enjoy being in it on a moment-to-moment basis. You can be glad you are in your body.

A lot of conversation these days revolves around teaching people how to feel happy in their bodies, how to ignore negative messages about body image and to be emotionally stable in their physical self. This growing trend is in response to an increasing number of people needing to feel comfortable in themselves. What we're talking about is the same idea, but it's a lot less in fashion because far fewer people have chronic pain than have chronic insecurities. Feeling *physically* comfortable and well in your body is just as important—if not more important—as being emotionally satisfied with it. You can't feel physically well all the time, but you can have a big impact on how often you do.

Feeling physically happy not only helps you through the bad patches, the actual physical pain, as it gives you something positive to hold onto and significantly ameliorates the negative psychological consequences of pain, but it also teaches the nervous system that there is another side to the coin. Your nervous system needs to know there is good stuff too; it can relax, it can be safe, it can feel well. You may feel bad now, but you can feel great later. Your body can feel good to you, and you can be comfortable in it. It's not just your consciousness that needs this information; your central nervous system does as well. Engaging in positive physical stimuli will desensitize you to pain and calm your nervous system on a long-term basis.

Neuroplasticity is the technical name for the brain's ability to change over time. Your brain has the ability to change its patterns and processes, both positively and negatively. You know this instinctively, as chronic pain is partly caused by learned patterns in how the body reacts. We're not going to go in depth here about the myriad causes and complications which come from the interaction between learned pain and ongoing pain as they relate to neuroplasticity, but if this is a topic you're interested in, I recommend the Australian Department of Health's pain health site for more information.[6] The good news we can take from this area of research is that the brain can relearn and retrain to form more positive connections between physical stimuli and your perception of pain. This is not pseudo-science or wishful thinking but proven actionable research that is applicable to your chronic pain issues. So encouraging and practicing positive physical stimuli is of primary importance. This can involve not just finding activities, like those listed above, that can feel good occasionally, but finding everyday pleasures as well.

Any number of seemingly minute things can feel great, but we just don't notice them. Sitting in a really comfortable chair can feel great, but we take it for granted. We don't notice. We only notice, perhaps, the absence of pain. An important part of retraining your nervous system comes not just from seeking out new and varied ways to stimulate positive physical responses, but also from teaching ourselves to be better observers of everything we touch and feel. What materials are your clothes made from? Are they soft, or scratchy? What kind of chair are you sitting on? Does it support you in all the right places, or have you automatically adopted the least-bad position and ignored it? Notice everything around you, how it feels, especially when it feels good. Washing your hands, brushing your hair, taking a shower; notice the little things consciously and be grateful for them. This may sound pedantic or cliché, but it truly helps. You have plenty of positive physical feelings in your body already; you just have to notice them and not let them be drowned out by the pain.

Some feelings that may, at first, be indistinguishable from pain or negative stimuli can, with practice, become positives. A good example of this is

6   "Neuroplasticity," Pain Health, last accessed May 15, 2019, https://painhealth.csse.uwa.edu.au/pain-module/neuroplasticity.

exercise; muscle tiredness and shortness of breath can be difficult and even concerning at first, but over time this feeling becomes associated with working hard, sleeping better, and the release of endorphins. You may find yourself seeking out activities that you once avoided because you have allowed yourself and your body to process, understand, and accept the feelings as natural and the consequences as good.

With time and constant engagement with your surroundings, the good, the bad, and the otherwise, your nervous system will learn to calm down. Not every tiny sensation will flip the alarm in your brain and tense you up. The ups and downs become smoother, more manageable. Your emotional connection to your body becomes stronger and more resilient. Your pain threshold will increase, and your ability to distinguish what is happening in your body will improve. Both you and your nervous system need this, so don't ignore it just because it's all the way back here in chapter 18!

Exercise:
Clearly Observe Your Own System

Pick one everyday activity that involves using your body. This should be something relatively simple and normal enough that you do it all the time without really thinking about it. This could be taking a shower, putting on your makeup, cuddling the dog; anything, but pick one.

Now, the next time you do this activity, pause beforehand. Notice how you are feeling in your body. Run through the five senses (sight, hearing, touch, taste, smell) before starting the activity. Register how you feel; what hurts? What is relaxed? Are you happy or grumpy or impatient? Don't judge, just notice.

Start doing your activity, no differently than usual—but throughout, notice everything. Notice how every part of it feels. For example, let's say you're taking a shower. Is the water warm or cold? How does it feel on your skin? Is it cascading down your head in gentle droplets or pummeling you with fierce streams of water? How does all of you feel? Run from your head to your feet, noticing each part of you, your crown, face, neck, throat, chest, shoulders, arms, hands, abdomen, belly, crotch, thighs, back, butt, knees, ankles, feet, toes. What can you feel in each different part of your body? How does moving around in the shower change this? Now you get the soap out; maybe you use a loofah or a scrubbing brush. What sensation does it cause against your skin? Are you looking at yourself as you wash? Can you smell any scents from the soap? Does the water pitter-patter against the shower door as it runs? Notice it all, without judgment or opinion, but just as it is. Do this throughout your process, changing nothing but your awareness.

Once you're done, sit down and think about how you feel now. What did you notice during your activity? Was there anything particularly pleasant or unpleasant? Do you feel better now, in yourself, or worse?

This practice can be applied to almost any activity and will help train you out of your just-get-through-it mode and enhance your ability to notice and accept physical pleasure.

Chapter 19

Support Groups

Even if you have the most supportive, empathetic family in the world, who are doing everything they possibly can to understand your chronic pain, it is not the same as someone who has been there, done that and lived through the same shit as you. It can't be. So do not underestimate the value of support groups. The opportunity and freedom to talk openly with people who are going through the exact same issue as you can be incredibly validating and cathartic, as well as practical. No one will know how to problem-solve like others in your same situation; you will always find novel ways to cope from people who've actually been there before.

"Support group" conjures up images of miserable, gray-looking people huddled about on metal folding chairs in the basement of some school or dingy community center, and understandably many people shy away from the concept of a) spending any time this way and b) talking frankly with total strangers about their most personal issues. But fear not! Most support groups have moved on from this 1970s stereotype, and many meet casually in coffee shops, restaurants or yes, sometimes, a public facility like a community center or mental health facility. Even these, though, are a far cry from the depressing picture many of us imagine. Genuinely kind, caring people set these groups up to help themselves and others and, if you give them a chance, they will help you. They'll help you process, vent, think, laugh, discover more information, and understand what you're going through, all in a safe and consequence-free environment that your loved ones can never provide, because of course you worry about their feelings and reactions in a way you just don't with strangers. You may even become friends with some of these people and have the joy of regular, open discussion about difficult chronic pain symptoms that become easier together.

There are a ridiculous number of support groups out there. If you live in a big city, there will almost certainly be one exclusively for people suffering from the specific illness you have. This kind of specificity is invaluable, but, for those in less populated areas, there are still very likely general support groups for chronic pain sufferers that will be of enormous benefit. Pushing yourself a little, giving it a go, may produce surprising results for you and your family. Remember, knowing that you have other support avenues will ease pressure from your loved ones too.

For the introverts who instinctively recoil from the notion of talking to strangers (or for the very busy), a less personal but still extremely useful method is accessing online support groups through pain websites, government resources, and non-profits, as well as on social media. You're probably on social media for at least part of your day anyway, so why not make it useful? There will definitely, absolutely be a specific support group online for whatever chronic pain you are experiencing, so look it up. The people in these groups are able to offer advice based on years of personal experience and will give you a great place to safely vent. Manageable, accessible support in a format you can digest, on a daily basis, is possible through online forums. And, as you become more expert in your own care, you will be able to pass on your knowledge to others. It can't hurt, it costs you nothing, and it will connect you with much-needed perspective and information on an ongoing basis.

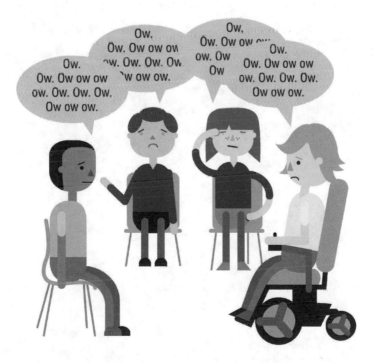

Lastly, don't forget professional bodies who offer valuable resources, connections with specialists, publications, and general support. There are a wide number of these, from the niche to the all-encompassing, and a curtailed list is below:

- American Academy of Pain Medicine—www.painmed.org

- American Pain Society—www.americanpainsociety.org

- American Pain Association—www.painassociation.org

- American Society of Regional Anesthesia and Pain Medicine— www.asra.com

- Canadian Pain Society—www.canadianpainsociety.ca

- Chronic Pain Association of Canada—www. chronicpaincanada.com

- International Association for the Study of Pain—www. iasp-pain.org

- The American Chronic Pain Association—www.theacpa.org

- US Pain Foundation—www.uspainfoundation.org

Exercise:
Find a Support Group

I'm not going to set an exercise suggesting you attend a local support group, because I know from personal experience how difficult this first step is and how unlikely people are to do it just because a book suggested it. No, instead I want you to do a very simple thing: go online and research support groups for chronic pain. If you have a specific pain-related disease, search for this. If you can't find something super specific, then find a general chronic pain management group. There are two options for this:

1. *In person.* If you're interested in meeting people in person, find the nearest group to you. See when they meet, conditions (if any) for attending, and where they are located. Now write this information down on a piece of paper, and put it away somewhere safe. It could be in your wallet, in a stack of papers on your desk, saved as a note on your phone—it doesn't matter. Just write it down.

2. *Online.* Many online groups will require you to "request to join," sign up for a newsletter, or simply perform a quick click of the "follow" button. Whichever group you choose, connect yourself to it online. You don't have to become an info-warrior right away; you can even hit the "snooze" button on seeing alerts or info from the group popping up in your feed. But make the connection, have that link so you can find it again quickly if you wanted to.

Simply knowing there are other people with similar chronic pain issues can be very comforting. Normalizing support groups is also important. One day you may feel a strong need for some extra support and then, hey! the first step is done, you know where to go or where to look already. There are no barriers or excuses. Maybe you will never feel that way; maybe you will lose this information or forget to check back in on it online; maybe you'll become an avid follower of other people's dilemmas online, but never take the step of engaging. None of these matter—the thing that matters is giving yourself the option.

Chapter 20

Planning for the Future

Okay, so you've done everything right. You've read this book, you've looked up your own information, you have open, candid relationships with your doctors and spouse and family, you take good care of yourself, et cetera, et cetera. But you're still in pain some of the time because that's what happens. There is no fix for that and, although you cope with it well and do everything you can, sometimes you feel awful and that's just all there is to it.

Knowing this, feeling the looming possibility in your body all day every day, can seriously affect your ability to plan for the future. How do you plan any big changes? How do you decide what you really want out of your life when the very first thought, for every single decision, is "Will it make me hurt more?" or "How will I know if I'll be able to?" Your judgment is slanted by the acceptance of your pain, by the urge to fight back, by the urge to take advantage of your good days while you can, by your guilt toward your loved ones, by the sheer immediacy of the need to get through each day… All of these impact the way you make big decisions and how you plan for your own future.

The reality of chronic pain conditions is that many worsen over time, hand in hand with our aging body's increasing immobility and decreasing ability to heal itself. Medications can become ineffective after continued use, family members become worn-down, bosses become less understanding, and the addition of the usual aches and pains people experience as they get older and settle into their bodies can tip you over the edge from coping to not.

You know this in your gut even if you don't like to think about it. This is how bodies work. Even if it hasn't started for you yet, even if it's a long way off or seems like a long way off, even if your chronic pain is the result of something that you expect to eventually clear up, aging will happen and your everyday experience of pain and suffering puts you in a much clearer position than many who spend their youth and middle age not worrying about the inevitability of their own bodies. Pain and age hits them like a slap to the face—it's a surprise—but for you it's been creeping about in your shadow for a long time. You're used to it.

One route isn't necessarily better than the other; those who are surprised by age get the joy of living (health-wise) carefree through their youth, and those who understand their body's fallibility well get the advantage of making the most of the time they have without wasting it. I hear that a lot from healthy people: "Blink and the time's gone...I woke up and I was suddenly old...I wish I'd known to think about that when I was young." You can think about what your pain and your health mean to your life now, while you are living it, rather than just at the end, and this is a blessing and a curse. It does cloud your decisions. It may bring some desires and hopes and issues into sharper focus. Or it may drive you to extreme conservatism, desperate to hold onto every last scrap of your body's capabilities by avoiding any risks at all. Both are understandable reactions.

Knowing that your pain may be with you through your life means that making smart choices now will significantly benefit you in the future. I don't just mean smart choices about career, although that is important, but who you surround yourself with, where you live, how you live, how you take care of yourself, planning for your financial future, whether to have kids or not, how many family members to support, long-term effects of medications, and much more. Even small changes or decisions, seemingly trivial, can make a huge difference to the future you. If you're buying your first house, you may not want to consider anything about your pain, but does it have a lot of stairs? Will you be able to manage them when your back goes out? If you want children and are the sole breadwinner in the family, what happens when you can no longer earn?

Maybe these issues don't come up for you; maybe you already know how to manage them. Maybe you're sure you'll always stay in the same state of physical health and so don't want to waste your time worrying about the future. Maybe you've just got your hands full managing today. Again, all of these possibilities are really normal, but be sensible. Know that your pain and your perception of your pain have an effect on your decisions. Be aware of this, consider it. How much of an effect do you want it to have? Are you letting it control your life, or are you balancing your reality with what you want? That's a hard thing to do, but it's the only way to take care of yourself physically and emotionally. Are you ignoring it and setting yourself up for disaster? Just be aware.

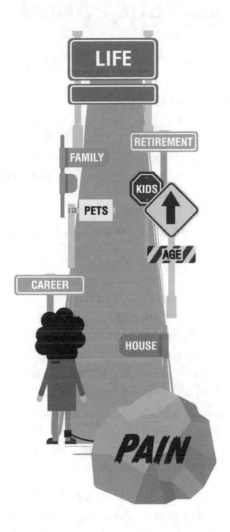

It's unrealistic to expect pain not to be a factor in your plans for the future, but be mindful of how big a factor you want it to be. You don't have to wallow, but you do have to be smart. And talk to your doctors—know the expected and likely progression of your health over time and as you age. More information never hurts in making plans, and knowing everything you can before planning for the future is just common sense.

Exercise:
Prioritize Your Future

Take a seat somewhere quiet and comfortable, with a pen and paper. Close your eyes. Imagine yourself five years from now. Imagine what you want, realistically, for yourself. Winning the lottery or marrying Taylor Swift are not what I mean. In your mind's eye, for yourself as you know you, as you actually are and where you live and who's around you, imagine what the best-case scenario would be for you in five years' time. Open your eyes, write it down. Are you with someone? Kids? What do you do for work? Where do you live? Note any differences from your life now; do you have certain hobbies or have you achieved something important to you, maybe a trip or schooling or a craft? Just jot them down in the order they occur to you.

Now close your eyes and do the same thing for future you, ten years from now. Again, this is best-case scenario but rooted in realism. Where do you want to be? If you're being realistic, it's probably a progression of the five-year expectation. Open your eyes and write down what you saw, noting anything different. Then repeat one final time, for old you. Imagine future you as a seventy- or eighty-year-old. Ignore the aches and pains you know you will feel at that age, and consider what you want your life to be in your twilight years (if you expect to reach them). Looking back on your life, what was important to you? What did you achieve that you were proud of, and what was a waste of your time? Again, write down as accurate a picture of this scene as you can.

Now look at what you've written and consider the life you have sketched for yourself, your actual self in your actual body. Yes, this may be the best-case scenario, and God knows any number of things might and probably will go wrong, but what's the ideal? Can you identify activities or people or work you are engaging with now that will be a waste of your time? Can you identify priorities for your life that you were unaware of, or that you have yet to start working toward?

List the top five differences or desires. Could be career, relationship, skills, anything. Then pick the most important one, just the one that sits in your chest and gives you that warm feeling thinking about it. If you're not doing it already, why not? Is it because of your physical limitations, or is it something more prosaic, like money or geography or family? Write down the barriers to this goal and then, one by one, address them. How can you get around them? What can you do to lessen the barriers? What steps can you take, now, to put you just one step closer to achieving this dream?

Doing this exercise can be valuable for anyone, but for those in chronic pain it provides the significant benefit of giving you a measure of control back over your life and empowering you, even in the midst of your pain. It's not about achieving every dream or always shooting for the moon, it's about doing everything you can to take steps forward when your body feels like it's pushing you back. You have power over yourself, your life, and your expectations. Use it; don't waste your precious energy and time on things that don't matter to you. Make the time you have, in pain or not, count for you. You are the only one living in and using your body, so what do you want it to be used doing?

Who Wants a Paint-by-Numbers Life Anyway?

I can hear the voices now that you've reached the end of this book, because they are the same voices that are in my head: "Isn't all of this legitimizing pain? Isn't all of this about allowing pain to control your life and change you? I don't want to change, I shouldn't have to."

Adapting is part of life, and adapting to your circumstances—whatever they may be—is necessary. This book is not about living without pain, it's about living with pain, every day. Pain is not the enemy. You may not like it, it may be difficult, but it is a part of your body, and so you need to accept it and take whatever steps you need to take to make your life better and easier with it. It's not always easy, but it's always worthwhile. Living with pain is normal; living with modifications and uncertainty and physical difficulties can also become normal. Everything covered in this book has fallen into one of two really broad categories to help you live through and past your pain: either normalizing what you need to do for you or understanding that the emotional and psychological effects of living in chronic pain are themselves perfectly normal. Learning both of these tenets as they apply to every part of your life is how you get past the barriers your pain throws in front of you. But it won't happen by accident, and it won't happen overnight.

All-or-nothing thinking is pernicious and damaging. You do not have to become an expert right away; you do not have to be able to tackle every exercise in this book in one go. It won't take a day, or even a year, but a lifetime of practice on how to live your life as best you can. All you can do is take one day at a time. Yes, that's a cliché, and no, that realization is not something you can force. It is only with time that you will be able to truly appreciate that the best you (or anyone) can do is take it one day at a time. It doesn't matter what happened yesterday or what will happen tomorrow, just do what you can today. That's all you can control. Try to manage your body for today. And then tomorrow, do the same thing. Just focus on the day. And do that, every day that you can, and every day it will become a little easier, and one day you'll realize you feel a little better, that you are so much stronger than you were, and that you're taking care of yourself without even realizing you're doing anything different.

The sheer volume of the ways in which pain can affect your life will often seem overwhelming, and this is true even if you've been living with it and managing it successfully for decades. It doesn't ever go away, it just becomes easier. There is no magic trick—it's repetition, repetition, repetition. And when you're overwhelmed, don't panic. It's a setback, just like any other. Go back to basics, and each time you do, it will be easier.

Almost every aspect of this book reflects almost every other aspect of this book. Boundaries are exercise are meds are resources are emotional management are everything. We have covered the same point in a hundred different ways, and the truth is that figuring out how to do just one of the self-care items listed will help you with all of them—because at the base of everything is the concept of putting your care first, without taking any blame or guilt for doing so. You are not your body but you are in your body, so it's your job to take care of it.

The fundamental truth is that there is no way to live your life exactly like everyone else, because everyone is managing, doing what they can, given their situation and needs and dreams. There is no right answer, no one solution, no paint-by-numbers methodology, for anyone, in pain or not. Everyone's life is full of compromises. Living with pain can feel like nothing but a series of crappy compromises, but, I promise you, almost every adult feels that way. What matters is how you deal with it. By following the steps in this book that speak to you, you are not transforming into a person without pain, but you are making self-care your new normal, and by doing this you open your life up to everything else in the world that's outside of your pain. You get more life by accepting what needs to be normal for you, then moving on.

Addendum:
For Caregivers

Just as your loved one has to learn how to live with chronic pain, you have to learn how to support and live with someone with chronic pain. Your job is hard, but don't be fooled—your loved one has it harder. You can always walk away, escape, have moments where you don't think about it. Your loved one can never escape their body. You can never know the suffocating certainty of their plight.

Your job as a caregiver is to walk the fine line between supporting your loved one and trying to do everything for them. It's between treating them as an equal and helping them when they need it (and helping, sometimes, without having to be asked). It's between having the perspective and detachment necessary to know when it's about their pain and when they're just being an ass. It's between empathy and smothering, detachment and distance, willingness to help and infantilization.

Is this an almost impossible task to do, every time, in every situation, regardless of how you are feeling and what's been happening and your own physical and emotional needs? Of course it is. No one is perfect, and no one can manage it all the time. Will you be blamed when you get it wrong? Maybe. No one said it was fair. No one said it would be easy. Being in pain isn't easy either, and your loved one is dealing with as much shit as you are. Your role—assuming you choose to accept it—is to offer the support and care that you can, while still taking care of yourself. Your job is to support your loved one, but be responsible for yourself. Your job is not to manage your loved one's pain, health, or emotional responses.

There are some practical ways to achieve this.

Actions to Support Your Loved One

1. Take On Physical Tasks around the Home

This could be cooking, cleaning, laundry, driving, shopping; find small ways to lighten their load. If this is not practical for you, don't do it. Taking on additional burdens if they will only overwhelm you helps nobody. But if there is something they find demanding or draining that you can easily take off their plate, do so. Talk to them about it; discuss what's trivial for you and hard for them and rebalance your division of labor accordingly.

2. Go with Them to the Doctor

Your support, even if it is silent throughout, can have a big impact on your loved one's ability to stick up for him- or herself. It also helps provide healthy perspective; your loved one may not always remember or know the extent of their symptoms, and you can, with their permission, be present to provide information that may help inform the doctor's medical opinion. Again, speak to your partner first and ensure they are comfortable with you doing this, but, if they are, be prepared to listen, support, and only provide your opinions if they are in direct contrast to your partner's and they have authorized you to do so. Butting into their doctor's appointment and walking all over them is not what we're suggesting here.

3. Problem-Solve with Them

If they are experiencing a problem, make it a shared problem. This doesn't mean you're going to fix it for them, but you can help them figure out what they want to do. You can support them and ensure they do not feel alone. Two heads are better than one, and something that may seem unsolvable to them may have an obvious solution to you. Be prepared to offer suggestions, but also be prepared for them to choose differently. As with any decision, if it is about them, they are the final arbiter, and you cannot be put out if they do not always follow your advice.

4. Rely on Your Loved One

Feeling useless is a common side effect of chronic pain. You can significantly reduce that by allowing your loved one to be a useful part of your life. Ask them to do things. Be sensible—maybe asking them to lift a sofa isn't the best idea—but ask them to pitch in. If they can't, that's okay, and you will probably already know what is reasonable to ask and what isn't, to help minimize their need to refuse you. There are a million tiny, non-physical things that they can still help you with, though, so ask them, even if you don't always feel like you *need* the help. They will gain an enormous sense of usefulness from knowing that your support for each other is mutual.

5. Reassure and Validate Them

Many chronic pain sufferers go a long time without being believed or listened to by medical professionals. Many still encounter people every day who do not listen or do not care that they are in pain, or simply think they are lazy, or stupid, or something else horrible and demeaning. Validate their expressions of pain, show them that you believe them. Reassure them that others' negative perceptions are flawed and not their responsibility.

6. Spend Time with Them Having Fun

It will benefit both of you hugely if you deliberately and frequently have fun together. This can be anything—gossiping, a movie, playing sports, a hobby—but it should be something you both enjoy doing together (or with others) and that isn't about their chronic pain. We all can so easily get stuck in coping mode, where everything is about managing pain or a health problem, and by doing so lose sight of living our lives. Enjoy each other, it will make you both feel a lot better.

7. Take Care of Yourself

This is vital. You are no help to your loved one if you are run-down, exhausted, sick, or overwhelmed. And they will only feel additional pressure to get through their pain whatever the cost to help you. You must take care of yourself. This means physically and emotionally. Being a caregiver is hard, and you are probably also working, dealing with stress, dealing with other relationships, taking on financial responsibilities, and who knows what else. But head down, blinkers on, just-get-through-it attitudes will not help in the long run. Below we have outlined some ways in which you can ensure you are taking proper care of yourself.

The physical and emotional burden of being a caregiver is enormous. Your primary responsibility is to take care of yourself, so you can better help your loved one. Taking care of yourself can mean:

- Taking time for yourself

- Socializing with friends and family

- Hobbies

- Exercise

- Managing your stress

- Proper sleep regimen

- Proper diet

- Asking your loved one for support when you need it

- Asking others for support and to share caregiving responsibilities

- Seeking out caregiver support groups for people in similar situations

Lessons to Learn

There are some lessons that are hard to learn for anyone but will come up frequently enough for you, as a caregiver, that you need to get used to them pretty quickly. This includes:

1. Knowing When to Do Nothing

This takes practice, as it goes against a lot of instincts, but there will be times when there is nothing you can do to help your loved one. You know this, they know this. But still, the urge is there to push, to suggest something else, to try to make it better. You want to make it better. You can't. You have to accept that. Constant suggestion or attempts to fix the unfixable will make your loved one feel unfixable; it is better and healthier for you both if you can say, "Yes, this sucks, I can't do anything to help, and now I feel useless and stupid" rather than repeatedly trying and failing to fix their problem.

2. Knowing You Are Not in Control

Ugh, this sucks, but neither of you are really in control of how their pain affects your lives, and trying to exert control over their pain is the same as trying to exert control over them. You can't do it, and they will resent you for trying.

3. Communicating

Neither of you is a mind-reader; just as your loved one is responsible for communicating to you how they feel, what they need, and what's going on, so are you. Holding back or attempts to protect them from additional stress or the effect their pain has on you does not work. They will know something is wrong and know you are not telling them, adding to their sense of alienation and uselessness. Treat them as they are, a reasonable adult with whom you can have open, frank conversations about all sorts of things.

4. Not Catastrophizing

Your loved one's pain may panic you, frighten you even, but panic never, ever helps. Listen to what they are saying and modulate your reaction. Panic and fear are your issues, not theirs, and discussing them with them is absolutely appropriate but not when they are in pain.

5. Choosing Your Moments

Some days are just going to be bad days. I'm sorry, but that's the way it is. Whether it's a bad pain day or your loved one is simply reacting to their pain in general through their mood, there will be some days when you cannot win. Reassurance is all you can offer on these days; let you loved one know you are there and you love them, and then leave everything else for another day.

6. Understanding There Are Some Things You Can't Understand

You do not know what it is like to be in their body, and you never can. Accept that there are some things you can't know, and trust your loved one in what they tell you without making endless, desperate attempts to understand before offering empathy or support. They do not have to validate themselves to you.

7. Recognizing the Person They Are Has Not Changed

Yes, they may be in chronic pain now, but they are still the same person. Tiptoeing around them, treating them differently, babying them, or ignoring them is not helpful.

8. It's Not about You

Do not personalize their pain. Do not personalize their emotional reactions to their pain. It is not about you, fundamentally, and you have to learn to live with that. Knowing when their state is caused by pain and not taking ownership of that will help you protect your emotional boundaries.

9. You Are Human Too

You can't fix it, you can't make it go away, you can't deal with it for them, you can't magically do everything by yourself, you can't be a robot. You are going to struggle. You are going to do absolutely the wrong thing sometimes. You're going to get angry. You are going to have to practice and sometimes, you just really won't want to. Won't want to practice, won't want to deal with them, won't want to deal with any of it. Believe me, they are having similar moments where they just don't want to, where they are angry and tired and frustrated and feel like nothing is getting better and want to give up. That's okay. It's not a reflection on them or you, just a sign that one or both of you needs a break and some perspective.

You do not have to do everything, and you do not have to do anything alone. Support and advice are available to you as a caregiver of someone in chronic pain. This is a challenging issue for anyone to have to deal with, and the most important thing you can do is to communicate with your loved one, openly and truthfully, about what they need, what you need, and how you can help and enjoy each other. You are only in it alone if you choose to be.

Summary of Important Lessons

Here are just some of the most important nuggets of wisdom from throughout the text; many of these can be used as affirmations.

- There is no magic bullet. You have to find a way to live in your body.

- All pain is real.

- You are not your pain.

- You must become your own best advocate.

- Your pain is more important than other people's expectations.

- Small changes are better than big ones.

- Always go at your own pace.

- Someone else's reaction to your boundaries has nothing to do with you.

- No is a complete sentence.

- You choose where to spend your energy.

- Having someone help you doesn't mean you've failed, it means you're not in it alone.

- There is no one right answer on how to behave or think, and what's right for you may change from day to day. Do what is right for you in the moment and forget the rest.

- What works for you is what works for you; do not waste energy defending it to others.

- No one is to blame for your pain, including yourself.

- It is okay to be anxious about your health, even if nothing has changed.

- Other people's coping with your pain cannot be, and is not, your problem.

- You do not have to ask for anyone's permission to take care of yourself. Be as weird as you like.

- Pain and suffering are not the same; you can live a life in pain without any suffering.

- Be realistic about what you can and cannot do, and build your work around that. Starting from anything else puts aspirations ahead of physical self-care.

- Filter your world of unrealistic expectations.

Afterword

Chronic pain is an extremely difficult subject to understand for all involved: difficult to treat for physicians and difficult to endure for those who suffer from it. *Taming Chronic Pain: A Management Guide for a More Enjoyable Life* just took you on a broad tour of the topic, starting with understanding the types of pain and ending with living life satisfactorily (if not happily) with proper pain management. She provides an honest account, mixed with humor, of numerous issues related to chronic pain, its understanding, and management.

It would be impossible for any physician to sit down and explain to every patient every aspect of pain, starting from its origin, and the numerous tools and therapies needed for living a life with pain. This book removes these barriers and fills the gap. It's easy to understand and follow, starting with a definition of pain which is crucial to understand, not only for patients, but also for providers. Many of us, especially patients, tend to perceive chronic pain as acute pain and expect treatment as such, which complicates the matter and leads to a multitude of issues.

One of the more important aspects for patients to understand is knowing their pain and explaining it to their doctors. It may be easy to explain to family members and friends (which may eventually lead you to losing them), but the important person to convey the information to is your physician. And the information needs to be accurate—not someone else's opinion or what you found online, but facts. Amy takes you through multiple issues, demonstrates how to talk to a doctor, and provides guidance that allows readers to absorb the information, in the process dispelling the myths and misunderstandings about pain and treatments.

As we all know, there is no miracle cure. Instead, Amy describes multiple types of treatments available and above all the importance of becoming your own advocate. As a physician, I always tell patients that managing pain depends 90 percent on them and 10 percent on the physician. To this end, Amy provides step-by-step information on making notes, talking to the doctor, going through the treatments, et cetera. She highlights the importance of exercise and discusses roadblocks many will face. She also explains the need for creating physical, emotional, and medical boundaries to account for the limitations that every aspect of pain enforce. She even provides an analysis of resource spending and utilizes economic theory!

Overall, it is crucial to have consistency and appropriate goals, an understanding of setbacks, and a knowledge of when give up. With all the treatments, it is important to use therapies which work, exercise, and retrain your nervous system, so you can continue with your life and live satisfactorily.

This book not only offers advice to patients, but also provides inherent advice for physicians in understanding the acute and chronic pain patient's perspective and how to manage them. I would recommend the book to all chronic pain sufferers or even those who have intermittent pain, their family members, and also the providers involved in managing chronic pain.

Laxmaiah Manchikanti, MD
Founder, Chairman and CEO of American Society of Interventional Pain
Physicians
Founder of the Pain Physician *journal*
Author of Interventional Pain Management *and 11 other works, including*
Interventional Techniques in Managing Chronic Pain

Acknowledgments

I have learned many lessons from my excellent and my terrible doctors over the years, and it is only with experience of both ends of the spectrum that I am able to appreciate the health care team I now have at my disposal. Special thanks to Dr. Melanie Beaton, for being the first doctor who treated me like a human being, to Dr. Sonya Mallone for always giving me as much time as I needed, and to Dr. Gerrie for her wise words. A big thank you also to Dr Morley-Forster, for her time, expertise and kindness, as well as her invaluable input to the book, and to Dr Manchikanti for his help. Lastly, I want to thank my dutiful husband, who has been through the ups and downs of living with pain and illness with me, learned with me, cried with me, gotten angry with me (and at me), and become my most fearless advocate and supporter. I would not be alive without your support through those first few difficult years.

Bibliography

There have been multiple texts, professionals, and websites who have helped provide information for this book. Below are just the main references:

1. *Living a Healthy Life with Chronic Conditions* by Kate Lorig, David Sobel, Virginia Gonzalez

2. *Critical Decisions* by Peter Ubel, MD

3. *Classifications of Pain* by Clifford J Woolf

4. *Building Better Boundaries* by Self Help Alliance

5. *Spoon Theory* by Christine Miserandino

6. *Mindfulness Efficacy* by Danny Penman

7. *The Anxiety & Phobia Workbook* by E. Borne

8. *You Are Not Your Pain: Using Mindfulness to Relieve Pain, Reduce Stress and Restore Well-Being* by Danny Penman & Vidyamala Burch

9. *The Mindfulness and Acceptance Workbook for Anxiety* by John P. Forsyth and Georg H. Eifert

10. *Radical Acceptance* by Tara Brach

11. *Life Disrupted* by Laurie Edwards

12. *How to Be Sick* by Toni Bernhard

13. *You Don't Look Sick* by Joy Selak PhD

14. *How to Live Well* by Toni Bernhard

About the Author

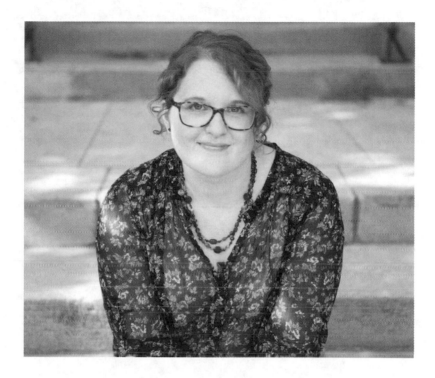

Amy is a passionate writer and scientist with an extensive history of living with, researching, and understanding pain disorders. Trained as a physicist, Amy has battled medical systems on two continents and has participated in, run, and is affiliated with multiple support and educational groups for the chronically ill. Her past writing ranges from long-form fiction to short-term educational pieces on healthcare, medical issues, and technology, and she has a wide online audience for these pieces. A Brit living in Canada with her husband and rescue greyhounds, she spends much of her free time volunteering with animal rescue, her local women's shelter, and mental health groups.

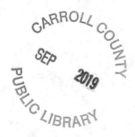